CONTENTS

Disclosure

Editors and authors of books and guidelines provided by the Oncology Nursing Society are expected to disclose to the readers any significant financial interest or other relationships with the manufacturer(s) of any commercial products.

A vested interest may be considered to exist if a contributor is affiliated with or has a financial interest in commercial organizations that may have a direct or indirect interest in the subject matter. A "financial interest" may include, but is not limited to, being a shareholder in the organization; being an employee of the commercial organization; serving on an organization's speakers bureau; or receiving research from the organization. An "affiliation" may be holding a position on an advisory board or some other role of benefit to the commercial organization. Vested interest statements appear in the front matter for each publication.

Contributors are expected to disclose any unlabeled or investigational use of products discussed in their content. This information is acknowledged solely for the information of the readers.

The contributors provided the following disclosure and vested interest information:

Deborah A. Boyle, RN, MSN, AOCNS®, FAAN: Pfizer, honoraria

Self-Healing Through Reflection: A Workbook for Nurses

by
Nancy Jo Bush, RN, MN, MA, AOCN®
Deborah A. Boyle, RN, MSN, AOCNS®, FAAN

Hygeia Media
An imprint of the Oncology Nursing Society
Pittsburgh, Pennsylvania

ONS Publications Department
Executive Director, Professional Practice and Programs:
Elizabeth M. Wertz Evans, RN, MPM, CPHQ, CPHIMS, FACMPE
Publisher and Director of Publications: Barbara Sigler, RN, MNEd
Managing Editor: Lisa M. George, BA
Technical Content Editor: Angela D. Klimaszewski, RN, MSN
Staff Editor II: Amy Nicoletti, BA
Copy Editor: Laura Pinchot, BA
Graphic Designer: Dany Sjoen

Library of Congress Cataloging-in-Publication Data
Bush, Nancy Jo.
 Self-healing through reflection : a workbook for nurses / by Nancy Jo Bush and Deborah A. Boyle.
   p. cm.
 Includes bibliographical references.
 ISBN 978-1-935864-13-4 (alk. paper)
 1. Nurses--Mental health. 2. Nurses--Job stress. I. Boyle, Deborah A. II. Title.
 RT86.B835 2012
 610.73--dc23

                                                                    2011028529

Publisher's Note
    This book is published by the Oncology Nursing Society (ONS). ONS neither represents nor guarantees that the practices described herein will, if followed, ensure safe and effective patient care. The recommendations contained in this book reflect ONS's judgment regarding the state of general knowledge and practice in the field as of the date of publication. The recommendations may not be appropriate for use in all circumstances. Those who use this book should make their own determinations regarding specific safe and appropriate patient-care practices, taking into account the personnel, equipment, and practices available at the hospital or other facility at which they are located. The editors and publisher cannot be held responsible for any liability incurred as a consequence from the use or application of any of the contents of this book. Figures and tables are used as examples only. They are not meant to be all-inclusive, nor do they represent endorsement of any particular institution by ONS. Mention of specific products and opinions related to those products do not indicate or imply endorsement by ONS. Web sites mentioned are provided for information only; the hosts are responsible for their own content and availability. Unless otherwise indicated, dollar amounts reflect U.S. dollars.
    ONS publications are originally published in English. Publishers wishing to translate ONS publications must contact ONS about licensing arrangements. ONS publications cannot be translated without obtaining written permission from ONS. (Individual tables and figures that are reprinted or adapted require additional permission from the original source.) Because translations from English may not always be accurate or precise, ONS disclaims any responsibility for inaccuracies in words or meaning that may occur as a result of the translation. Readers relying on precise information should check the original English version.

Printed in the United States of America

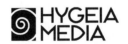

An imprint of the Oncology Nursing Society

PREFACE

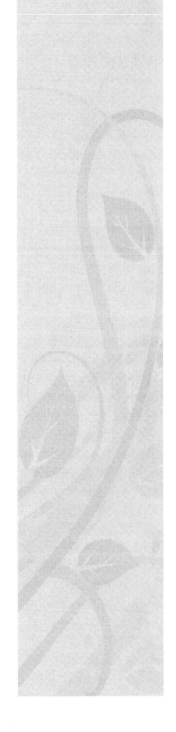

Medical professionals are held in high esteem, especially nurses, who are generally admired for their altruism and selflessness. Competence in caring is widely accepted as a foundational value that distinguishes nursing from other professions (Rhodes, Morris, & Lazenby, 2011). By nature, nurses are gifted healers. Their words communicate hope, their touch extends compassion, and their presence, even in the most painful of circumstances, offers comfort and assurance.

Qualities of trust, commitment, honor, integrity, and courage are but a few that nurses exemplify. By applying these values in their work, across all healthcare settings, nurses are the backbone of quality patient care. They are the liaison between the medical and interdisciplinary teams—doctors, social workers, physical therapists, and chaplains. Nurses are the major providers of patient care. The Agency for Healthcare Research and Quality acknowledged that the majority of what happens to a patient in the hospital setting involves nursing care. Every individual who has entered the healthcare system can offer testimony that it was the nurse who stood at the front line of care.

Yet, the labor of nursing is stressful. McNeely (2005) noted that because stress is an assumed cost of doing nursing work, it often is interpreted as the individual's responsibility to counter it. Why, then, is it that the very professionals who render care for others find it so difficult to nurture themselves? Some simply call this entity *self-care*; we prefer to acknowledge it as *self-healing*.

This phenomenon has significance across the entire trajectory of nursing care within multiple settings. Although it is most often discussed in palliative, pediatric, and critical care, the absence of self-nurturance is a shared experience within all specialties. It is also relevant to the varied roles in nursing—bedside and advanced practice nurses, nurse educators and researchers, nurse managers and executives. Many words have been applied, often interchangeably, to this lack of self-care: *burnout, compassion fatigue, secondary and traumatic stress, nurse grief,* and others. Yet, a caveat is in order. While the theoretical constructs behind these terms are not interchangeable, the ill effects on the individual nurse often are. We are vulnerable to become wounded healers.

Nurses' self-care and healing are long-overlooked attributes of professional longevity and fulfillment. The purpose of this workbook is twofold. First, we want to help nurses positively reaffirm the initial commitment and energy that typified their motivation to choose nursing as a profession. Second, we aspire to help nurses gain insight and awareness into the professional and personal stressors that can negatively affect them along their journey of caregiving. By using the information, exercises, assessment tools for reflection, and suggestions for workplace interventions provided in this book, nurses can formally counter the current paradigm of emotional depletion. Once nurses can identify their risks for problematic coping and lack of self-healing, they can use the knowledge and skills imparted in this workbook to find their way back to a place of renewal, safety, and resilience. We hope that these travels will aid our colleagues in sanctioning the value of caring, not only for patients and their loved ones, but also for themselves.

Fondly,

Nancy Jo Bush
Deborah A. Boyle

References

McNeely, E. (2005). The consequences of job stress for nurses' health: Time for a check-up. *Nursing Outlook, 53,* 291–299. doi:10.1016/j.outlook.2005.10.001

Rhodes, M.K., Morris, A.H., & Lazenby, R.B. (2011). Nursing at its best: Competent and caring. *Online Journal of Issues in Nursing, 16*(2). doi:10.3912/OJIN.Vol16No02PPT01

Chapter

1

BURNOUT

Introduction

Nursing is a challenging profession characterized by a significant number of stressors. These include demanding work environments, time pressures, and workload. *Burnout* is a term used to describe environmental conditions of the workplace that contribute to an employee's feelings of disempowerment, abandonment, and stress. Maslach (1993) defined burnout as *job stress.* Burnout is a cumulative condition that results in physical, emotional, and mental exhaustion. Conditions that contribute to workplace frustration are most commonly related to inadequate staffing ratios and a lack of positive reinforcement such as staff break time and educational and administrative support. The nurse becomes "burned out" related to feeling a lack of support, lack of leadership or role modeling, and the inability to be a change agent within the work environment. Essentially, the nurse may feel "stuck" and immobilized—tied to a job because of fear of change or issues related to finances or benefits. Feelings of powerlessness to change the work situation may ensue.

The concept of burnout has been studied since the 1970s and has focused on the relationship that people have with their work environment. Burnout is "a prolonged response to chronic emotional and interpersonal stressors on the job and is defined by the three dimensions of exhaustion, cynicism, and inefficacy" (Maslach, Schaufeli, & Leiter, 2001, p. 397). Exhaustion comes in the form of being emotionally drained, cynicism is reflected

Notes

in the depersonalization of others, and inefficacy is related to feelings of marginal productivity accompanied by feelings of low achievement. The risks of burnout include diminished caring and a profound sense of demoralization (Leiter & Laschinger, 2006; Maslach, 1993). People who are considered burned out become overly emotionally involved in their work, overextend themselves by juggling too many responsibilities at once, feel overwhelmed by the emotional demands placed upon them by other people in their work environment, and, in extreme cases, are overwhelmed by interpersonal relationships outside the workplace (Stebnicki, 2008).

Behavioral symptoms of burnout may range on a continuum from detachment from patients and fellow caregivers to anger and acting out, to apathy. Extreme feelings of burnout may lead to behavioral problems outside of the workplace such as interpersonal problems, fatigue and sleep disturbances, withdrawal, and isolation. Psychological domains related to burnout may include anxiety, depression, and the risk of compassion fatigue, vicarious traumatization, and, ultimately, secondary traumatic stress disorder. Inevitably, both the associated feelings and the behavioral manifestations of burnout negatively affect the nurse's work function. The nurse feels overextended, ineffective, and stressed. The inherent risks of burnout to the environment include a decreased quality of nursing care and high rates of staff dissatisfaction and turnover.

Maslach et al. (2001) identified six areas of the work setting that contribute most to the context of burnout: workload, control, reward, community, fairness, and values.

- **Workload:** Excessive workload is linked directly to the exhaustion associated with burnout. Nurses also may expend additional emotional energy if not prepared adequately for the work required or if experiencing feelings of incompetence.
- **Control:** If nurses do not feel control over the workload or feel that insufficient resources are available to enact the quality caregiving to which they aspire, then self-esteem is negatively affected.
- **Reward:** In many settings where nurses are overworked and have limited resources, they also begin to feel underrecognized

for their hard work and effort. Lack of social rewards for work well done is associated with feelings of inefficacy.

- **Community:** Nurses must feel a sense of belonging or collegiality with others in the work setting along with shared values and goals. If role conflict or hostility exists among peers, then the important element of social support is lacking.
- **Fairness:** If nurses perceive unfair treatment of themselves or others, this can contribute to mistrust and cynical feelings about the workplace and leadership.
- **Values:** It is important that nurses feel a match between personal and workplace values, or they may become resentful if constraints cause behaviors that they find to be unethical or morally wrong (see Chapter 7).

The organizational stressors leading to burnout must be recognized in light of the era of managed care and healthcare reform. Many nurses at the bedside feel that their profession has become a job and that the focus of their work environment has changed from one of caring for and healing the sick to a business focus— do more with fewer resources and in less time. Within the construct of burnout, the nurse is left with feelings of helplessness and hopelessness. In the literature, a major demographic factor that contributes to burnout is age: the younger and more inexperienced the nurse, the higher the risk of burnout (Espeland, 2006). Idealistic, highly motivated, and highly empathic nurses are the first to burn out, as does a bright flame by virtue of its intensity (Larson, 1993; Larson & Bush, 2006). The organizational risks of burnout are listed in Figure 1.

Figure 1. Organizational Risks of Burnout
Burnout: The progressive loss of idealism or the professional's unrealistically high expectations concerning his or her work given a clinical, social, and organizational environment that is perceived as resistant to change.   • Diminished job performance   • Decreased job effectiveness   • Impaired personal and social functioning   • Resignation; high staff turnover   • Termination

Notes

REFLECTION

Burnout Self-Test*

Answer the following questions using this numeric scale:

1 = Not at all   2 = Rarely   3 = Sometimes   4 = Often   5 = Very often

Do you feel run down or drained of physical or emotional energy?   ____

Do you find that you are prone to negative thinking about your job?   ____

Do you find that you are harder or less sympathetic with people than perhaps they deserve?   ____

Do you find yourself getting easily irritated by small problems or by your coworkers and team?   ____

Do you feel misunderstood or unappreciated by your coworkers?   ____

Do you feel that you have no one to talk to?   ____

Do you feel that you are achieving less than you should?   ____

Do you feel under an unpleasant level of pressure to succeed?   ____

Do you feel that you are not getting what you want out of your job?   ____

Do you feel that you are in the wrong organization or profession?   ____

Are you becoming frustrated with parts of your job?   ____

Do you feel that organizational politics or bureaucracy frustrates your ability to do a good job?   ____

Do you feel that there is more work to do than you practically have the ability to do?   ____

Do you feel that you do not have time to do many of the things that are important to doing a good quality job?   ____

Do you find that you do not have time to plan as much as you would like to?   ____

Total   ____

Score Interpretation	
Score	**Comment**
15–18	Little sign of burnout here.
19–32	Little sign of burnout here, unless some factors are particularly severe.
33–49	Be careful—you may be at risk for burnout, particularly if several scores are high.
50–59	You may be at severe risk for burnout—seek advice; take action.
60–75	You may be at very severe risk for burnout—seek advice; take action.

*This is not a scientifically based test but just questions to provide reflection. There are many intervening variables influencing stress and burnout.

Note. From "Burnout Self-Test," by Mind Tools. Retrieved from http://www.mindtools.com/pages/article/newTCS_08.htm. Copyright by Mind Tools Ltd. Adapted with permission.

The American Association of Critical-Care Nurses (AACN, 2005) identified six essential standards that are vital for ensuring healthy work environments. These standards represent evidence-based practice and relationship-centered principles of interdisciplinary care. The standards are supported by the American Nurses Association's (2001) *Code of Ethics for Nurses*. These standards can guide nurse leaders and healthcare organizations to ensure safety and quality care for patients and safe practice and respect for nurses. The standards comprise skilled communication, true collaboration, effective decision making, appropriate staffing, meaningful recognition, and authentic leadership. They provide a framework for nursing practice that prevents burnout and the risks that may occur along the continuum of compassion fatigue and secondary traumatic stress disorder (McKinley, 2007). McKinley (2007) discussed the components of the AACN standards.

- **Skilled communication:** Effective communication skills are as essential as competent clinical skills. The two are interdependent in nature. *Skilled communication* is defined as a two-way dialogue in which members of the interdisciplinary team think and make decisions together. Skilled communication includes verbal, nonverbal, and written communication and ensures respect and civility to the nurse. "Intimidating behavior and deficient interpersonal relationships lead to mistrust, chronic stress, and dissatisfaction among nurses" (McKinley, 2007, p. 246).
- **True collaboration:** Interdisciplinary staff members must support true collaboration that ensures all members of the team are respected for their unique knowledge and competence. Mutual concern for quality care is shared in true collaborative practice.
- **Effective decision making:** Research supports that the majority of physicians do not utilize nurses effectively in decision making and that nurses feel powerless to change their work environment. As the mainstay professionals who assess, diagnose, intervene, and evaluate patient care, nurses must be included in patient decision-making practices. If not, a vital link is lost along the patient care continuum.
- **Appropriate staffing:** Increased workloads without appropriate staff resources threaten patient safety and nurse satisfaction. Healthcare environments must adequately assess patient acuity

Notes

Notes

levels and resources on an ongoing basis and investigate staffing models that meet the needs of patients and nurses alike.

- **Meaningful recognition:** Nurses must be recognized for the value that each brings to the institution. Recognition for work well done also ensures nurse recruitment and retention.
- **Authentic leadership:** "Nurse leaders must fully embrace the imperative of a healthy work environment, authentically live it, and engage others in its achievement" (McKinley, 2007, p. 251). The AACN standards noted that nurse leaders play a pivotal role in nurse retention, and yet they themselves are at risk for burnout resulting from a lack of educational preparation, coaching, or mentoring for their roles (AACN, 2005).

REFLECTION

What advantages does your work setting provide? _____

_____

_____

_____

What do you do best in your work setting? _____

_____

_____

_____

What do your managers see as your strengths? _____

_____

_____

_____

What behaviors and feelings do you have that translate into quality care? _____

_____

_____

_____

_____

(Continued on next page)

REFLECTION *(CONTINUED)*

What can you improve in your work setting?_____

_____

_____

_____

What are good opportunities facing you in the future? _____

_____

_____

_____

What professional organizations have you joined to support your professional goals?_____

_____

_____

_____

Note. Based on information from Corley, 1995.

Interventions

Because nurses are routinely considered vulnerable to burn-out, they must consciously plan to counter the negative sequelae of work-related stress. Additionally, burnout may be contagious (Bakker, Le Blanc, & Schaufeli, 2005). The negative attitudes, behaviors, and complaints of colleagues can be communicated from one nurse to another. A major intervention is to know that understanding the signs of burnout and taking action can lead to professional growth. The first step is for the nurse to identify what he or she can and cannot do to change the work environment. Knowledge is empowerment, and knowing what steps can be taken can lead to feelings of empowerment (Corley, 1995).

The following interventions can help to prevent burnout and inherent moral distress (Corley, 1995; McKinley, 2007).

- **Don't blame.** A major response to burnout is to blame oneself or others. Blaming oneself may include feeling that peers and colleagues are able to cope with the circumstances within the job setting, whereas you are unable to cope effectively. Unfor-

Notes

tunately, this line of thinking negatively affects self-esteem and feelings of self-efficacy. Burnout leads to feelings of isolation, and projecting blame onto others will further contribute to behaviors of withdrawal. Guilt and blame also are perpetuating and lead to a vicious negative cycle.

- **Take action.** Taking action is the most effective way to decrease feelings of burnout. Action can begin by stepping back and reflecting upon those circumstances that have led to feeling burned out in the work environment. Self-knowledge is empowering and will help to decrease feelings of helplessness. Reflect upon what actions may be taken to change the circumstances that are causing the most stress. Trusting other colleagues with feelings related to burnout is important. Is there someone you can trust to talk to and share your feelings with? Are there colleagues that share the same frustrations and who might be able to brainstorm regarding changes that can be made in the work environment in order to assist and support each other? The support of a formal mentor or preceptor has been cited as an invaluable resource to counter stress (Barnard, Street, & Love, 2006).

- **Take control.** Identify what you can and cannot do to change your work circumstances—and focus on what you do have control over. For example, how you decide to take action to change your own behaviors is an important initial step toward change. Strengthen your own assertiveness skills and learn to say "no" when appropriate. Know your own triggers and find ways to manage them.

- **Seek advice.** Another vehicle is to think about helpful changes that you can bring to the table and then speak to a professional colleague who is in a position to help you make the change. For example, a nurse manager or advanced practice nurse (APN) may be available for support. Educational resources, time management changes, or administrative change may decrease the feelings of burnout among all nurses experiencing it in your work setting. Working together as a team will enhance everyone's feelings of hopefulness that yes, things can be changed within the setting and that working together can make it happen. Think of things that you can improve versus things to avoid or ignore. A staff meeting could be held to discuss ways to improve teamwork and the delivery of care. Monthly support groups could be initiated—not for whining about problems but for evaluating the outcomes of implemented changes. Joining professional organizations in a specialty area is also an important means of gaining insight and ideas for how to keep moving forward in these times of healthcare changes and challenges. Taking part in professional organizations will also keep you up to date on evidence-based practice, in turn increasing your feelings of self-efficacy and competence.

- **Reframe.** Reframe your work and the work setting in a more positive light. Ask yourself, "What advantages does my work setting provide for me and my patients?" Think about your own strengths and what others perceive your strengths and contributions to be.

- **Set goals.** Reflecting upon your professional and personal goals is another positive problem-solving step to take. Maybe the setting you are working in does not nurture these goals, and it is time to take your talents to a new and different setting. Transitioning from inpatient to outpatient care or changing specialty practice can often rekindle enthusiasm and the desire to learn. Think about the good opportunities that are ahead in your work and your life, which may help you feel "unstuck." By reframing the circumstances that you find yourself in and setting new goals, you may be pleasantly surprised that you are doing your best with limited time and resources, most importantly contributing to the quality of care your patients receive. Focus on the positive. Make sure that the job is a good fit for your values and expertise. When there is a mismatch in job fit, the risk of burnout increases.

- **Practice self-care.** Basic self-care includes exercise, adequate rest and sleep, and good nutrition. Preventing burnout includes these interventions and also may include challenging yourself to a higher level of spirituality and insight. You can do this through reflective work: meditation, guided imagery, yoga, journaling, and other activities. Treat yourself with massage therapy or, if needed, interpersonal therapy. Find support from relationships outside of the work setting—support systems that can listen to

Notes

Notes

your concerns objectively and provide feedback. Identify something to look forward to each day, in or out of the work setting. This may be quiet moments in a garden or taking time to walk with a close friend or loved one.

- **Be resilient.** Human beings are resilient souls. People who demonstrate hardiness and resilience are less prone to burnout. *Resilience* is the ability to confront immeasurable challenges with strength and fortitude. It includes self-confidence and self-assurance, seeing oneself as a survivor. Resilient individuals experience the same difficulties and stressors as everyone else; they are not immune or hardened to stress. Yet, resilient people have learned how to deal with life's challenges. They are set apart by their optimistic and hardy attitude.

Summary

Burnout is a syndrome of emotional exhaustion, depersonalization, and feelings of reduced personal accomplishment in one's job. When the nurse's emotional resources are depleted, the nurse is no longer able to give of himself or herself on a psychological level. Burnout can contribute to negative and cynical attitudes and a reduced sense of personal accomplishment. Strategies against burnout include organizational change in addition to the nurse reflecting upon avenues to change the circumstances leading to burnout.

Case Study

Mary was exhausted. Every morning when the alarm rang and she swung her legs over the side of her bed, they felt like lead weights. She wondered why she felt more tired on days she had to work. She dreaded going to work. Mary had worked on the same medical-surgical unit since she was a new graduate nurse 10 years ago. In the beginning, she loved her job and the community of nurses with whom she worked. Back then, she always thought to herself, everyone worked as a team. The staff shared similar values in quality care, and they took the time to socialize outside the work setting. As time passed and health care changed, Mary experienced unsettling changes on her unit. Her friends began to leave, some pursuing other positions and a few colleagues quitting nursing entirely. Staffing seemed to get cut each year as people left and positions were not replaced. At one time, there was an APN assigned to the unit. The APN was always available to consult on challenging patients, and monthly patient rounds or educational meetings were held. When the cost-cutting began, the APNs were some of the initial positions to be cut. Seldom was there a nurse colleague to call upon to consult with challenging patients or families, and Mary couldn't remember the last educational meeting that took place on the unit. She found herself so exhausted at night that she couldn't even find the energy to read her journals, so she stopped ordering them. As time passed, Mary did the minimum to keep up her necessary continuing education units for relicensure.

Mary woke up exhausted and came home exhausted. She always felt irritable and found herself snapping at her coworkers and her family members. When she tried to reflect upon why she went into nursing in the first place, she couldn't remember. She became cynical about her profession and hopeless that anything could change to make it better. Often she felt remorse and guilt that she was not giving quality care to her patients because she did not have the time or supportive resources to do it.

Discussion

Mary was definitely displaying physical, psychological, and behavioral symptoms of burnout. She woke up every morning fatigued and exhausted and dreaded going to work. Her behaviors manifested in irritability and cynicism. Mary also felt hopeless that she or her work setting could change. As her friends left and resources became scarce, Mary felt guilt related to the lack of care she believed her patients received and also was remorseful that she found herself feeling as she did.

In Mary's case, a few problem-solving, action-oriented steps could be taken. In lieu of the now-absent APN position, Mary could search out a new role model or mentor within her setting. This could be a fellow colleague, a nurse manager, or even another interdisciplinary team member. It was important for Mary to feel that she was supported in her care setting and that a trustworthy person was available to consult regarding difficult or challenging situations. Mary could also suggest changes that would benefit her and her coworkers in keeping up to date in their practice. Mary could suggest a weekly journal club to discuss articles related to medical-surgical nursing. The journal club also would contribute to a sense of belonging and teamwork among the staff. Another valuable resource for Mary would be to attend more community educational opportunities and join a professional organization to help her feel like a valuable part of the nursing profession. These latter resources also could help Mary find solutions to patient cases she found challenging, and she would then feel valued for her contributions when she brought this education back to her work setting.

References

American Association of Critical-Care Nurses. (2005). *AACN standards for establishing and sustaining healthy work environments: A journey to excellence.* Retrieved from http://www.aacn.org/WD/HWE/Docs/HWEStandards .pdf

American Nurses Association. (2001). *Code of ethics for nurses with interpretive statements.* Silver Spring, MD: Author.

Bakker, A.B., Le Blanc, P.M., & Schaufeli, W.B. (2005). Burnout contagion among intensive care nurses. *Journal of Advanced Nursing, 51,* 276–287. doi:10.1111/j.1365-2648.2005.03494.x

Barnard, D., Street, A., & Love, A.W. (2006). Relationships between stressors, work supports, and burnout among cancer nurses. *Cancer Nursing, 29,* 338–345.

Corley, M.C. (1995). Moral distress of critical care nurses. *American Journal of Critical Care, 4,* 280–285.

Espeland, K.E. (2006). Overcoming burnout: How to revitalize your career. *Journal of Continuing Education in Nursing, 37,* 178–184.

Larson, D.G. (1993). *The helper's journey: Working with people facing grief, loss, and life-threatening illness.* Champaign, IL: Research Press.

Larson, D.G., & Bush, N.J. (2006). Stress management for oncology nurses: Finding a healing balance. In R.M. Carroll-Johnson, L.M. Gorman, & N.J. Bush (Eds.), *Psychosocial nursing care along the cancer continuum* (2nd ed., pp. 587–601). Pittsburgh, PA: Oncology Nursing Society.

Leiter, M.P., & Laschinger, H.K.S. (2006). Relationships of work and practice environment to professional burnout: Testing a causal model. *Nursing Research, 55,* 137–146.

Maslach, C. (1993). Burnout: A multidimensional perspective. In W.B. Schaufeli, C. Maslach, & T. Marek (Eds.), *Professional burnout: Recent developments in theory and research* (pp. 19–32). Washington, DC: Taylor & Francis.

Maslach, C., Schaufeli, W.B., & Leiter, M.P. (2001). Job burnout. *Annual Review of Psychology, 52,* 397–422. doi:10.1146/annurev.psych.52.1.397

McKinley, M.G. (2007). AACN standards for establishing and sustaining healthy work environments: A journey to excellence. Appendix C. In M.G. McKinley (Ed.), *Acute and critical care clinical nurse specialists: Synergy for best practices* (pp. 243–254). Philadelphia, PA: Elsevier Saunders.

Stebnicki, M.A. (2008). *Empathy fatigue: Healing the mind, body, and spirit of professional counselors.* New York, NY: Springer.

Recommended Reading

Emold, C., Schneider, N., Meller, I., & Yagil, Y. (2011). Communication skills, work environment and burnout among oncology nurses. *European Journal of Oncology Nursing, 15,* 358–363. doi:10.1016/j.ejon.2010.08.001

Leiter, M.P., & Maslach, C. (2005). *Banishing burnout: Six strategies for improving your relationship with work.* San Francisco, CA: Jossey-Bass.

Maslach, C. (2003). Job burnout: New directions in research and intervention. *Current Directions in Psychological Science, 12,* 189–192. doi:10.1111/1467-8721.01258

Maslach, C., & Leiter, M.P. (1997). *The truth about burnout: How organizations cause personal stress and what to do about it.* San Francisco, CA: Jossey-Bass.

Maslach, C., & Leiter, M.P. (2008). Early predictors of job burnout and engagement. *Journal of Applied Psychology, 93,* 498–512. doi:10.1037/0021-9010.93.3.498

Poghosyan, L., Clarke, S.P., Finlayson, M., & Aiken, L.H. (2010). Nurse burnout and quality of care: Cross-national investigation in six countries. *Research in Nursing and Health, 33,* 288–298. doi:10.1002/nur.20383

Internet Resources

LIVESTRONG, "Preventing Burnout": www.livestrong.com/article/14719-preventing-burnout

Maslach Burnout Inventory: www.mindgarden.com/products/mbi.htm

Mind Tools, Burnout Self-Test: www.mindtools.com/stress/Brn/BurnoutSelfTest.htm

Notes

COMPASSION FATIGUE

Introduction

Joinson (1992) discussed the concept of *compassion fatigue* (CF) resulting from the overwhelming stress faced by nurses. Joinson's definition of CF incorporated the construct of burnout but heightened the awareness of the *empathic engagement* that is inherently involved in the work of those in the caring professions: nurses, doctors, ministers, counselors, and others. Nurses who experience CF may experience helplessness in response to the stress they feel in watching patients go through a devastating illness or trauma (Yoder, 2010). Figley (1995, 2002) stated that CF was the cost of caring for others in emotional pain. An understanding of CF and the inherent coping strategies necessary to prevent it may help to avoid negative effects on the personal lives of nurses, enhance their ability to carry out their work effectively, improve the quality of patient caregiving, and prevent nurses from leaving the profession (Yoder, 2010).

Compassion has been defined as a complex phenomenon that enables caregivers to hold and sustain emotional equilibrium while holding patients' despair in one hand and their hope in the other (Lewin, 1996). The components of compassion are empathy and devotion, responsibility, nurture, and preservation (Valent, 2002). To be truly compassionate, nurses must be resilient and steadfast in their personal beliefs and values. Compassion is the foundational value of the nurse's work, and compassion gives nursing its soulfulness and healing powers (Lewin, 1996). Stamm (1999) stated, "The capacity for compassion and empathy seems to be at the core of our ability to do the work and at the core of our ability to be wounded by the work" (p. xv). Compassion and empathic engagement can be a double-edged sword—an honorable personality trait but also a side of vulnerability (Larson & Bush, 2006). Yoder (2010) discussed that CF has been closely linked with burnout, yet they have been envisioned as two separate entities. Burnout is related to goal setting and achievement, whereas CF is related to a rescue-caretaking response (Valent, 2002). Burnout has been viewed as the frustration, helplessness, and diminished morale that occur when the nurse fails to reach his or her goals. CF results in feelings of guilt or distress when the nurse feels that he or she cannot save the patient from harm (Valent, 2002; Yoder, 2010).

Which nurses are at highest risk for CF? Nurses who are idealistic, highly motivated, and committed are at greatest risk to experience burnout and CF. It is the idealistic, highly empathic caregivers who often are the first to burn out (Larson, 1993; Larson & Bush, 2006). Figley (1999) stated that those caregivers who have an enormous capacity for feeling and expressing empathy tend to be more at risk for compassion stress and fatigue. Young, inexperienced nurses who feel ill-prepared for high-stress environments, for heavy caseloads, and for caring for the extremely ill have been identified as vulnerable to burnout and CF as well. Cumulative, unresolved losses also put nurses at risk, along with the feelings of disappointment and despair that often occur simultaneously with feelings of inefficacy and low self-esteem.

The experience of CF is thought to transcend the cumulative exhaustion that is typical of organizational burnout. Figley (1999) discussed variables that make individuals more prone to CF and empathy fatigue in their work with traumatized people. First, being empathic is a key factor in the transmission of traumatic material from the primary source to the secondary "victim." Second, individuals who have experienced some traumatic event in their own lives are at greater risk for CF, and unresolved trauma of the individual can be activated by the traumatic experiences of the patient. Finally, similar to burnout, CF also may have a contagion effect that can be transmitted to the nurse's support system—coworkers, family, and friends (Bakker, Le Blanc, & Schaufeli, 2005; Figley, 1999).

REFLECTION

Professional Quality of Life Scale (ProQOL)
Compassion Satisfaction and Fatigue—ProQOL Version 5 (2009)

When you nurse people, you have direct contact with their lives. As you may have found, your compassion for those you nurse can affect you in positive and negative ways. Below are some questions about your experiences, both positive and negative, as a nurse. Consider each of the following questions about you and your current work situation. Select the number that honestly reflects how frequently you experienced these things in the <u>last 30 days</u>.

1 = Never   2 = Rarely   3 = Sometimes   4 = Often   5 = Very often

_____1. I am happy.

_____2. I am preoccupied with more than one person I nurse.

_____3. I get satisfaction from being able to nurse people.

_____4. I feel connected to others.

_____5. I jump or am startled by unexpected sounds.

_____6. I feel invigorated after working with those I nurse.

_____7. I find it difficult to separate my personal life from my life as a nurse.

_____8. I am not as productive at work because I am losing sleep over traumatic experiences of a person I nurse.

_____9. I think that I might have been affected by the traumatic stress of those I nurse.

_____10. I feel trapped by my job as a nurse.

_____11. Because of my nursing, I have felt "on edge" about various things.

_____12. I like my work as a nurse.

_____13. I feel depressed because of the traumatic experiences of the people I nurse.

_____14. I feel as though I am experiencing the trauma of someone I have nursed.

_____15. I have beliefs that sustain me.

_____16. I am pleased with how I am able to keep up with nursing techniques and protocols.

_____17. I am the person I always wanted to be.

_____18. My work makes me feel satisfied.

_____19. I feel worn out because of my work as a nurse.

_____20. I have happy thoughts and feelings about those I nurse and how I could help them.

_____21. I feel overwhelmed because my workload seems endless.

_____22. I believe I can make a difference through my work.

_____23. I avoid certain activities or situations because they remind me of frightening experiences of the people I nurse.

_____24. I am proud of what I can do to help.

_____25. As a result of my nursing, I have intrusive, frightening thoughts.

_____26. I feel "bogged down" by the system.

(Continued on next page)

REFLECTION *(CONTINUED)*

____27. I have thoughts that I am a "success" as a nurse.

____28. I can't recall important parts of my work with traumatized patients.

____29. I am a very caring person.

____30. I am happy that I chose to do this work.

Self-scoring directions, if used as self-test

1. Be certain you respond to all items.
2. Go to items 1, 4, 15, 17, and 29 and reverse your score. For example, if you scored the item 1, write a 5 beside it. We ask you to reverse these scores because we have learned that the test works better if you reverse these scores (1 = 5; 2 = 4; 3 = 3; 4 = 2; and 5 = 1).

What is my score and what does it mean?

To find your score on *Compassion Satisfaction,* add your scores on questions 3, 6, 12, 16, 18, 20, 22, 24, 27, and 30. Compassion satisfaction is about the pleasure you derive from being able to do your work well.	**Sum of My Compassion Satisfaction Questions**	**So My Score Equals**	**My Level of Compassion Satisfaction**
	22 or less	43 or less	Low
	Between 23 and 41	Around 50	Average
	42 or more	57 or more	High
To find your score on *Burnout,* add your scores on questions 1, 4, 8, 10, 15, 17, 19, 21, 26, and 29. Burnout is one of the elements of compassion fatigue. It is associated with feelings of hopelessness and difficulties in dealing with work or in doing your job effectively.	**Sum of My Burnout Questions**	**So My Score Equals**	**My Level of Burnout**
	22 or less	43 or less	Low
	Between 23 and 41`	Around 50	Average
	42 or more	57 or more	High
To find your score on *Secondary Traumatic Stress,* add your scores on questions 2, 5, 7, 9, 11, 13, 14, 23, 25, and 28. The second component of compassion fatigue is secondary traumatic stress (see Chapter 4). It is about your work-related, secondary exposure to extremely or traumatically stressful events.	**Sum of My Secondary Traumatic Stress Questions**	**So My Score Equals**	**My Level of Secondary Traumatic Stress**
	22 or less	43 or less	Low
	Between 23 and 41	Around 50	Average
	42 or more	57 or more	High

The construct of CF can be best understood as the second step of a continuum beginning with burnout and ending in secondary traumatic stress disorder. CF emanates from a state of compassion discomfort to compassion stress and finally to compassion fatigue, which, if not addressed in its earliest phases, can permanently alter a nurse's compassion ability (Coetzee & Klopper, 2010).

The concepts will be differentiated in the next few chapters, but the importance is that nurses, nurse leaders, and other interdisciplinary members, including physicians, identify the symptoms of burnout at an early stage so as to prevent the development of deeper wounding that may occur along the continuum of helping others who are in emotional pain. CF is inherently the "natural, predictable, treatable, and preventable unwanted consequence of working with suffering people," and the concepts that parallel CF are burnout and countertransference (Figley, 1999, p. 4).

Countertransference is the emotional reaction to the patient by the nurse. It is the distortion of judgment on the part of the nurse resulting from the nurse's life experiences and is associated with an unconscious response to the patient's transference of emotional, and in some cases physical, pain. Why is the concept of countertransference important in nursing? If the nurse overidentifies with a patient or attempts to meet his or her own needs through a patient, unbiased care cannot be ensured and professional boundaries become blurred. The patient's pain becomes the nurse's pain, and vice versa.

Nurses who work with patients with chronic and life-threatening illnesses, the dying, and the bereaved are especially vulnerable to the effects of countertransference and CF. Dying patients touch nurses deeply in many ways. Death and dying makes the nurse more aware of personal losses and arouses existential anxiety in the nurse's personal death awareness (Stebnicki, 2008). During empathic engagement, especially in traumatic cases, there can be an unconscious absorption of the patient's journey. *Empathy* is a form of intense listening that is facilitated by the nurse in a personal relationship with the patient (Stebnicki, 2008). Empathic listening is involved in all communication skills that nurses

Notes

employ to assess the patient's experience: clarifying the patient's perspective, restating the intended meaning of the experience to the patient, reflecting understanding of the feelings being expressed, and then always summarizing the patient's experience to move the journey forward. The nurse uses these empathic listening skills with the patient, family members, physicians, and other interdisciplinary staff involved in the patient's care. It is not surprising then that the nurse may feel an overidentification with the patient's feelings and concerns, often finding a symbolic or parallel experience. This also can be viewed as a form of vicarious traumatization, which contributes to both burnout and CF.

Interventions

"Balanced" empathy is the key to avoiding the end points of the continuum—emotional overinvolvement with patients and families and the other extreme of emotional exhaustion or burnout (Larson & Bush, 2006). Compassionate care for the self is vital for the nurse to not just survive but to thrive in the profession and in the attainment of personal goals. Nurses must prepare their minds, bodies, souls, and spirits to become resilient in working with patients at intense levels of interpersonal functioning (Stebnicki, 2008). Resiliency may be an innate personality characteristic, yet it also can be learned (Bush, 2009). Nurses learn about resiliency and courage from their patients when they transform adversity into challenge and find hope in the most hopeless of situations (Larson & Bush, 2006). Nurses are highly motivated and committed caregivers. They must engage in activities that comfort, restore, and rejuvenate empathic caring and presence. "Only when nurses take time to heal themselves can they be truly available to aid in the healing of others" (Bush, 2009, p. 27).

Self-care strategies can appear straightforward: exercise, adequate rest and sleep, nutrition, relaxation, and use of support systems. When a nurse suffers from burnout and CF, however, physical and emotional exhaustion often prevents the nurse from taking the time to initiate these measures. Highly empathic nurses also may subconsciously feel that taking the time for self-care is selfish if it takes away from work-related projects or valuable time with family and friends outside of the work setting. This represents a different but similar double-edged sword—a personality trait of selfless giving but a vulnerable point of self-starvation (Larson & Bush, 2006). Welsh (1999) outlined six strategies for avoiding CF.

- **Practice responsible selfishness.** An internal belief of the nurse is that his or her needs are secondary to those of others. Engaging in activities to recharge and renew personal energy is necessary to remain responsive to the needs of others.

- **Separate work from home.** The demands of work and home often are in conflict because of stressors and time constraints. Transitional strategies to leave work at work may include using commute time to decompress, carrying out an exercise regimen after work, or practicing meditation and guided imagery. A healthy barrier can minimize the interactions between personal and professional stressors.

- **Develop positive support groups.** Nurses should surround themselves with individuals who are willing to listen, empathize, and problem solve with mutual understanding. This can be in the form of peers and colleagues. Relationships unrelated to similar work environments can provide objective viewpoints on a distressing situation. If a nurse is suffering from severe burnout or CF, then group or individual psychotherapy is indicated.

- **Refuse to be a victim.** Dwelling on the realities of managed care and healthcare reform, which the nurse has limited control over, causes many nurses to feel helpless, thus exacerbating negative feelings. Welsh (1999) advised, "Dwelling on that reality obscures another reality: personal freedom in our behavioral, cognitive, and affective responses" (p. 184).

- **Remember to laugh.** The old adage applies here: "Laughter is good medicine." Hearty and sustained laughter has been found to relieve stress and boost immune response. Carry out activities that promote laughter, such as social events with friends, movies, and yes, even finding the ability to laugh at our own gaffes.

Notes

Notes

- **Redefine success.** Setting personal goals helps to decrease burnout and CF by identifying a match between the nurse's professional goals and the practice setting. For high achievers, a sense of personal failure is a major contributing factor to CF. Nurses should reframe their expectations and value each small but very significant contribution they make for each patient they care for on a daily basis. Welsh (1999) stated that if nurses do not end the day feeling successful, then they have probably been looking in the wrong places. The key to self-care may surpass straightforward strategies and instead rely upon the nurse's spirituality and sense of self-worth in a broader perspective (see Chapter 6). Interventions that tap into the spiritual nature of the nurse's work can be integrated into the clinical setting and into personal activities.

Summary

Situations that nurses have described as contributing to CF and burnout include those related to patient care, organizational problems, and personal issues (Yoder, 2010). Patient care issues may range from caring for gravely ill and traumatized patients to situations in which the nurse feels helpless (e.g., caring for a patient with a poor prognosis yet who is receiving aggressive treatment). Work-related stressors include high acuity, poor staffing ratios, high census, heavy patient assignments, and overtime. Personal issues have been described as including inexperience, inadequate energy, and close personal identification with patients.

Coping strategies that help nurses to prevent or recover from CF have been identified as work-related and personal strategies (Yoder, 2010). Effective coping includes *taking action* to manage or change the work environment. Countertransference issues play a major part in contributing to CF. A common strategy for preventing countertransference issues is to change the personal engagement that the nurse develops with patients (Yoder, 2010). The end goal is for nurses to develop healthy, therapeutic relationships with patients and yet protect themselves by developing appropriate emotional boundaries and practicing self-care behaviors.

Case Study

Whenever someone smiled at Sally and she smiled back, all she could feel was an empty, drained heart. Sally had worked in the emergency department for almost five years now. Before this job, Sally worked in the cardiac care intensive care unit (ICU). She changed positions five years ago when she was beginning to feel drained and apathetic about her staff position in the ICU. Initially, working in the emergency department provided Sally with learning experiences that motivated her in her career. There were no educational programs to prepare her for emergency department nursing, so she essentially learned on the job.

Sally worked in a trauma emergency department, so every day she faced emergent cases that were life-threatening: car accidents, gunshot wounds, abuse, rape, and assault. During each shift, Sally and others would joke to each other as they asked, "What are we in for tonight?" When Sally began working in the emergency department setting, she found this unknown to be an exciting challenge. She never knew what or who would be coming through the doors. Twelve-hour shifts passed quickly, often with no time for breaks or even mealtimes. Sally and her peers ran on pure energy fueled only by their own adrenaline. Sally would leave a shift thoroughly physically exhausted and often would spend the next day sleeping late, catching up on errands, and caring for her two young children. There was never a time to even reflect upon the numerous physical and emotional demands that she faced each day.

What had been Sally's naturally happy and smiling personality was now more reactive than sincere. The emotional and physical exhaustion she had felt when she left the ICU slowly crept back and affected her spirits. Yet, she was totally taken aback by her recent feelings of worry and despair. She hadn't seen it coming. Sally no longer looked forward to her work but instead dreaded going, and no matter how busy she was, the 12 hours often seemed like days. She found herself irritable and tense, and, for the first time in her life, she felt a sadness that she could not pinpoint. For years, Sally had worked hard to save her patients against all odds and had many success stories. But during those times, she would be emotionally present for family members and friends who were

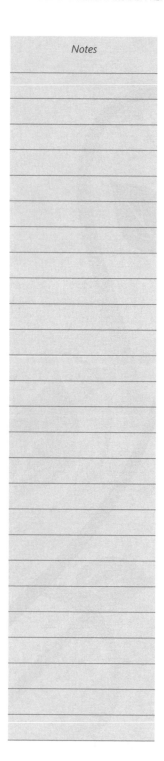

thrown into the throngs of grief. For many years, her caring and compassionate nature carried her through these difficult times. Sally could even feel compassion for the worried mother of a child with a sore throat and fever and patiently walk her through what was a benign case compared to the frightening happenings that often occurred.

Tonight there had been an unexpected death in the emergency department—an innocent young man caught in gang crossfire. Sally felt the overwhelming trauma in her body and mind, and at times she feared that her emotions would become uncontrollable. Somehow she was able to support the family, handle their grief, and assist them with the decisions that had to be made regarding funeral preparations. Yet, Sally could not reach her car fast enough when her shift ended. Rolling tears blurred her eyesight, and when she finally locked herself in the car, she was engulfed with shaking sobs and wrenching grief. What was wrong?, Sally asked herself. Why was she feeling this way? And she couldn't get home fast enough to check on her sleeping children in their beds.

Discussion

It is evident that Sally was initially suffering from burnout before her transfer from the ICU to the emergency department. Her strategic move was positive in that the new clinical setting challenged her and warded against the long-term stressors that often cannot be ignored when working in settings for extended periods of time. Whether Sally ever fully recovered from burnout is not known, but she most likely carried some unresolved losses and feelings into her new clinical setting. She also transferred from one high-anxiety setting to another, facing life-threatening situations, losses, and grief.

No doubt Sally was experiencing symptoms of CF. Unbeknownst to Sally, the feelings of exhaustion and sadness had been building up until she was dreading going to work. No longer did she feel excited or challenged, and the time at work dragged on because of her physical and emotional exhaustion. Sally ignored her self-care needs both at work and at home. She didn't take breaks during 12-hour shifts or mealtimes on the busiest of days. At home Sally felt her personal needs were secondary to her young children. She didn't feel she could take time to exercise or visit with friends when three days per week she couldn't spend quality time with her children or husband. She was totally drained, so much so that she had yet to recognize the signs and symptoms.

Sally first needs to acknowledge how physically and emotionally drained she has become from her job. She also must identify the signs of her psychological isolation from family and friends who could offer her support. Once Sally realizes that she is feeling the responsibility of rescuing all of her suffering patients— from the young child with the sore throat to the young man with the gunshot wound—she can work toward reinforcing all the positive contributions she makes to patient and family quality of life and redefine the meaning of her work. In doing so, she can acknowledge that she cannot prevent the loss and suffering of others but can certainly ameliorate some of their pain. In addition to redefining the outcomes of her work, Sally needs to identify self-care strategies that would help to build her physical and emotional resources.

Notes

REFLECTION

Answer the following open-ended questions.

What signs of CF does Sally display? _____
_____
_____
_____

What initial self-care strategies would you suggest for Sally? _____
_____
_____
_____

What strategies would you suggest that may be helpful for the ER staff? _____
_____
_____
_____

Notes

References

Bakker, A.B., Le Blanc, P.M., & Schaufeli, W.B. (2005). Burnout contagion among intensive care nurses. *Journal of Advanced Nursing, 51,* 276–287. doi:10.1111/j.1365-2648.2005.03494.x

Bush, N.J. (2009). Compassion fatigue: Are you at risk? *Oncology Nursing Forum, 36,* 24–28. doi:10.1188/09.ONF.24-28

Coetzee, S.K., & Klopper, H.C. (2010). Compassion fatigue with nursing practice: A concept analysis. *Nursing and Health Sciences, 12,* 235–243. doi:10.1111/j.1442-2018.2010.00526.x

Figley, C.R. (1995). Compassion fatigue as secondary traumatic stress disorder: An overview. In C.R. Figley (Ed.), *Compassion fatigue: Coping with secondary traumatic stress disorder in those who treat the traumatized* (pp. 1–20). New York, NY: Brunner/Mazel.

Figley, C.R. (1999). Compassion fatigue: Toward a new understanding of the costs of caring. In B.H. Stamm (Ed.), *Secondary traumatic stress: Self-care issues for clinicians, researchers, and educators* (2nd ed., pp. 3–28). Lutherville, MD: Sidran Press.

Figley, C.R. (2002). Introduction. In C.R. Figley (Ed.), *Treating compassion fatigue* (pp. 1–14). New York, NY: Brunner-Routledge.

Joinson, C. (1992). Coping with compassion fatigue. *Nursing, 22,* 118–120.

Larson, D.G. (1993). *The helper's journey: Working with people facing grief, loss, and life-threatening illness.* Champaign, IL: Research Press.

Larson, D.G., & Bush, N.J. (2006). Stress management for oncology nurses: Finding a healing balance. In R.M. Carroll-Johnson, L.M. Gorman, & N.J. Bush (Eds.), *Psychosocial nursing care along the cancer continuum* (2nd ed., pp. 587–601). Pittsburgh, PA: Oncology Nursing Society.

Lewin, R.A. (1996). *Compassion: The core value that animates psychotherapy.* Northvale, NJ: Jason Aronson.

Stamm, B.H. (1999). Preface to the first edition. In B.H. Stamm (Ed.), *Secondary traumatic stress: Self-care issues for clinicians, researchers, and educators* (2nd ed., pp. xv–xviii). Lutherville, MD: Sidran Press.

Stebnicki, M.A. (2008). *Empathy fatigue: Healing the mind, body, and spirit of professional counselors.* New York, NY: Springer.

Valent, P. (2002). Diagnosis and treatment of helper stresses, traumas, and illnesses. In C.R. Figley (Ed.), *Treating compassion fatigue* (pp. 17–37). New York, NY: Brunner-Routledge.

Welsh, D.J. (1999). Care for the caregiver: Strategies for avoiding "compassion fatigue." *Clinical Journal of Oncology Nursing, 3,* 183–184.

Yoder, E.A. (2010). Compassion fatigue in nurses. *Applied Nursing Research, 23,* 191–197. doi:10.1016/j.apnr.2008.09.003

Recommended Reading

Aycock, N., & Boyle, D. (2009). Interventions to manage compassion fatigue in oncology nursing. *Clinical Journal of Oncology Nursing, 13,* 183–191. doi:10.1188/09.CJON.183-191

Boyle, D.A. (2006). Desperate nursewives [Editorial]. *Oncology Nursing Forum, 33,* 11. doi:10.1188/06.ONF.11

Boyle, D.A. (2011). Countering compassion fatigue: A requisite nursing agenda. *Online Journal of Issues in Nursing, 16*(1), Manuscript 2. doi:10.3912/OJIN.Vol16No01Man02

Gentry, J.E. (2002). Compassion fatigue: A crucible of transformation. *Journal of Trauma Practice, 1*(3/4), 37–61. doi:10.1300/J189v01n03_03

Hooper, C., Craig, J., Janvrin, D.R., Wetsel, M.A., & Reimels, E. (2010). Compassion satisfaction, burnout, and compassion fatigue among emergency nurses compared with nurses in other selected inpatient specialties. *Journal of Emergency Nursing, 36,* 420–427. doi:10.1016/j.jen.2009.11.027

Levine, S. (2005). *Unattended sorrow: Recovering from loss and reviving the heart.* Emmaus, PA: Rodale.

Najjar, N., Davis, L.W., Beck-Coon, K., & Doebbeling, C.C. (2009). Compassion fatigue: A review of the research to date and relevance to cancer-care providers. *Journal of Health Psychology, 14,* 267–277. doi:10.1177/1359105308100211

Potter, P., Deshields, T., Divanbeigi, J., Berger, J., Cipriano, D., Norris, L., & Olsen, S. (2010). Compassion fatigue and burnout: Prevalence among oncology nurses [Online exclusive]. *Clinical Journal of Oncology Nursing, 14,* E56–E62. doi:10.1188/10.CJON.E56-E62

Rothschild, B. (with Rand, M.L.). (2006). *Help for the helper: The psychophysiology of compassion fatigue and vicarious trauma.* New York, NY: W.W. Norton & Company.

Sabo, B.M. (2006). Compassion fatigue and nursing work: Can we accurately capture the consequences of caring work? *International Journal of Nursing Practice, 12,* 136–142. doi:10.1111/j.1440-172X.2006.00562.x

Showalter, S.E. (2010). Compassion fatigue: What is it? Why does it matter? Recognizing the symptoms, acknowledging the impact, developing the tools to prevent compassion fatigue, and strengthen the professional already suffering from the effects. *American Journal of Hospice and Palliative Medicine, 27,* 239–242. doi:10.1177/1049909109354096

Walton, A.M.L., & Alvarez, M. (2010). Imagine: Compassion fatigue training for nurses. *Clinical Journal of Oncology Nursing, 14,* 399–400. doi:10.1188/10.CJON.399-400

Internet Resources

Compassion Fatigue Awareness Project, Compassion Fatigue Self-Test: www.compassionfatigue.org/pages/CompassionFatigueSelfTest.html

Professional Quality of Life Scale: www.proqol.org/ProQol_Test.html

Self-Care Academy, Compassion Fatigue: http://self-careacademy.com/sca/?page_id=152

Notes

VICARIOUS TRAUMATIZATION

Introduction

*V*icarious traumatization is a concept that refers to a transformation in the nurse's inner experience resulting from empathic engagement with patients' traumatic experiences (Pearlman & MacIan, 1995). Differentiated from compassion fatigue, vicarious traumatization changes the worldview or inner cognitive schema of the nurse experiencing it. For example, after working for prolonged periods of time with death and dying patients, the nurse may begin to view the world as unfair and fate as unjust to those who are vulnerable to suffering. The experience of vicarious traumatization goes beyond the emotional and psychological effects of empathy that contribute to compassion fatigue (Blair & Ramones, 1996). The nurse experiencing vicarious traumatization ultimately questions the meaning and purpose of life (Sinclair & Hamill, 2007).

As defined by Saakvitne and Pearlman (1996), the construct of vicarious traumatization can be best understood by the following: "When we open our hearts to hear someone's story of devastation or betrayal, our cherished beliefs are challenged and we are changed" (p. 25). Vicarious traumatization is viewed as the human consequence of both caring for and facing the reality of traumatic experiences in others. The specific impact of vicarious traumatization is a result of the interaction between the *situation* (e.g., the work setting, the cultural, social, and political context of the trauma) and

Notes

the *personality* of the nurse (e.g., prior trauma experiences, coping style, prior life experiences). Vicarious traumatization represents the profound loss of what has been familiar—safety, control, predictability, and protection (Saakvitne & Pearlman, 1996). Vicarious traumatization implies changes in the nurse's way of experiencing oneself, others, and the world. The changes that occur are cumulative across time and helping relationships (Pearlman & MacIan, 1995).

Vicarious traumatization is based upon a self-development and interpersonal model termed *constructivist theory*. The construct of vicarious traumatization delineates how prolonged exposure to traumatic experiences can negatively affect psychological development. Understanding the components of this theory helps to explain its impact on the nurse's inner self. Saakvitne and Pearlman (1996) and Sinclair and Hamill (2007) outlined the components of the self that are affected by vicarious traumatization, depicted by the following.

- **Frame of reference.** The *self* incorporates a frame of reference that includes one's sense of identity, worldview, and spirituality. This frame of reference influences people's perception of themselves, the world, and the relationships and experiences within it. Nurses experiencing vicarious traumatization may feel disconnected from their sense of identity and less grounded in their belief system. Behavioral indicators may include feelings of being overwhelmed, angry, anxious, and irritable or having crying outbursts. They may feel alone and in despair, and feelings of numbness may set in. The nurse may ask, "Why don't I feel sad for my patients anymore? I just cannot care anymore."

- **Self-capacities.** A *sense of self* is influenced by an inner balance that allows the nurse to manage strong feelings, feel entitled to be alive and deserving of love, and to have the empathy to care for others. Vicarious traumatization creates a state of disconnection and can leave one feeling alone, questioning whether he or she deserves to feel loved or happy. The risk of these feelings is that it is difficult to hold hope for traumatized patients when the nurse cannot hold onto faith and self-assurance.

- **Ego resources.** These are skills in *self-awareness*, such as insight and the ability to take on the perspective of another, including empathy. Ego resources support the use of willpower, initiative, and personal growth. Nurses experiencing vicarious traumatization may be unable to make sound decisions, fail to set limits, and overextend responsibilities. Their boundaries may become blurred, causing feelings of resentment, failure, and emotional exhaustion.

- **Psychological needs and cognitive schemas.** Saakvitne and Pearlman (1996) defined the five major psychological needs outlined in constructivist theory: safety, esteem, trust, control, and intimacy. Cognitive schemas are these psychological needs, such as safety, reflected in what the nurse holds true about his or her self. Meeting these needs also supports self-esteem and trust in others. Nurses suffering from vicarious traumatization may have decreased feelings of self-efficacy and control. Working with traumatized patients also may unravel beliefs about one's own safety and the safety of loved ones. Vicarious traumatization causes changes in the schemas of safety, trust, and control. Nurses may lose trust in coworkers and those in leadership positions and may develop a sense of powerlessness. Losing perspective and hope is a risk of vicarious traumatization. Losing trust in others can make the nurse feel misunderstood and isolated.

- **Memory and perception.** Memory is encoded along the dimensions of cognitive, visual, emotional, somatic, sensory, and behavioral input. Nurses who have vicarious traumatization will have fragmented memories and perceptions of a traumatic experience (e.g., the untimely death of a young patient). Flashbacks may occur with panic or terror. Boelen and Huntjens (2008) used the term *intrusive imagery* to describe the sudden and unintentional reemergence of autobiographical incidents that elicit stress. Saakvitne and Pearlman (1996) stated that these symptoms parallel post-traumatic stress disorder (PTSD) symptoms and are termed *secondary traumatic stress disorder* (STSD).

These symptoms can include psychological numbing, avoidance of reminders of the traumatic event, flashbacks, and nightmares. Figure 2 depicts the signs and symptoms of vicarious traumatization.

Personal characteristics may increase the risk of vicarious traumatization. These include a personal trauma history, the meaning

Notes

Notes

of traumatic life events to the nurse, psychological and interpersonal style, professional development, and current stressors and support systems. Characteristics of the work setting that may contribute to vicarious traumatization include the patient population and intensity of care required, stressful patient needs and behaviors, and the sociocultural context (Pearlman & MacIan, 1995). Emergency department nurses who are continually exposed to accidents, abuse, neglect, and premature death are particularly vulnerable to vicarious traumatization (Lavoie, Talbot, & Mathieu, 2011). Having a personal trauma history is a powerful risk factor for vicarious traumatization (Pearlman & MacIan, 1995).

Figure 2. Cognitive Changes and Symptoms Associated With Vicarious Traumatization

Changed Worldview
- Disrupted frame of reference
- Changes in identity, worldview, and spirituality
- Diminished self-capacities
- Impaired ego resources
- Disrupted psychological needs and cognitive schemas
- Alterations in memory, perception, and sensory experiences

Symptoms
- No time or energy for oneself
- Disconnection from loved ones
- Social withdrawal
- Cynicism
- Generalized despair and hopelessness
- Nightmares

Note. From *Transforming the Pain: A Workbook on Vicarious Traumatization* (p. 40), by K.W. Saakvitne and L.A. Pearlman, 1996, New York, NY: W.W. Norton & Company. Copyright 1996 by the Traumatic Stress Institute/Center for Adult & Adolescent Psychotherapy LLC. Reprinted with permission.

REFLECTION

Signs of Vicarious Traumatization

As a result of your work with patients and families, what *changes* have you noticed in the following areas of your life and beliefs?

Frame of Reference

My identity and beliefs about myself: Who am I? _____

_____

My view of and beliefs about the world: How do I see it? _____

_____

My spirituality (sense of connectedness and meaning, faith): How has it changed? _____

_____

My work motivation: Are my reasons for doing this work different from when I started it? _____

_____

Self-Capacities: My Inner Sense of Balance

How am I managing strong feelings? _____

_____

Can I keep loved ones in my mind and know they care about me? _____

_____

Do I feel worthwhile, deserving, and lovable? _____

_____

Ego Resources: Using My Resources on My Own Behalf

Am I using my resources to make good decisions in personal and professional relationships (self-protective judgment, boundaries)? _____

_____

Am I using my resources to know myself better (introspection) and to keep growing? _____

_____

(Continued on next page)

REFLECTION *(CONTINUED)*

Basic Psychological Needs and My Beliefs About Them

1. *Safety* for myself and those I love
   Do I feel reasonably safe? _____

   Do I believe my loved ones are safe? _____

2. *Esteem* for myself and other people
   Am I proud of who I am? _____

   Do I believe others deserve respect? _____

3. *Trust* in myself and other people
   Do I believe I can trust my own judgment? _____

   Do I feel I can trust or depend on others? _____

4. *Control* in my life and over others
   Do I believe I have control over my life? _____

   Do I believe I can influence others' behaviors? _____

5. *Intimacy* and closeness with myself and others
   Do I believe I am good company for myself? _____

   Do I believe I can be close to others? _____

Changes in Sensory Experiences: Intrusive Imagery and Sensations

Do I experience more nightmares? _____

Do I have intrusive thoughts about my own or others' safety? _____
_____

Do I experience intrusive images or sensory experiences? _____
_____

Am I reactive to triggers connected to my patients' experiences? _____
_____

How is my body showing stress or responding differently? _____
_____

Have I noticed changes in my experience of self, such as numbing, depersonalization, hypersensitivity, or increased somatization? _____
_____

Note. From *Transforming the Pain: A Workbook on Vicarious Traumatization* (pp. 57–59), by K.W. Saakvitne and L.A. Pearlman, 1996, New York, NY: W.W. Norton & Company. Copyright 1996 by the Traumatic Stress Institute/Center for Adult & Adolescent Psychotherapy LLC. Reprinted with permission.

Interventions

Addressing vicarious traumatization is "an ethical imperative" (Saakvitne & Pearlman, 1996, p. 49). It is both a personal and organizational responsibility to initiate preventive measures. Although it is difficult, nurses need to know their own vulnerabilities for burnout, compassion fatigue, and vicarious traumatization. It is important to protect oneself from depletion and self-harm. Seeking counseling or other therapeutic interventions for emotional distress is part of self-care and mental health. Saakvitne and Pearlman (1996) discussed two measures for counteracting vicarious traumatization. The first is to *address the stress* inherent in vicarious traumatization by focusing on self-care activities. The second is the need to *transform* the negative beliefs, despair, and loss of meaning associated with the demoralization and loss of hope that occur with vicarious traumatization.

Management of the stress and demoralization encompassed by vicarious traumatization can begin with changes within the organizational structure of the workplace. Similar to prevention of burnout, organizational and leadership strategies are necessary to ameliorate, if not prevent, the causative factors contributing to vicarious traumatization. Organizations can foster an environment in which stress is normalized and accepted. This helps the nurse to not feel alone and isolated. Resources such as clinical education and supervision, peer support groups, and multidisciplinary support, including pastoral care, can all prove beneficial. Saakvitne and Pearlman (1996) asserted that work setting variables such as type and number of patients, their diagnoses, traumas, and the social, political, and cultural context will all interact with the nurse's experiences and vulnerability to vicarious traumatization. The risks of burnout caused by organizational stressors discussed in Chapter 1 apply to vicarious traumatization as well.

Saakvitne and Pearlman (1996) divided self-care strategies into three categories: self-care, nurturing oneself, and escaping. *Self-care* is defined as finding balance, maintaining a healthy lifestyle, setting limits, and connecting with others. *Nurturing* is defined as treating oneself with gentleness and focusing on comfort, relaxation, and play. *Escape* is defined as activities that allow one to for-

Notes

get about the stressors of work by engaging in fantasy or getting away from painful feelings (e.g., entertainment, time with family and friends, vacation). Activities alone are not viewed as infusing the *meaning* into life that is required to heal from vicarious traumatization. Carrying out meaningful activities such as playing with one's grandchildren or participating in community building is best to combat vicarious traumatization. The negative beliefs, cynicism, and despair associated with vicarious traumatization must be challenged by the meaning infused into self-care, nurturing oneself, and escape activities. Saakvitne and Pearlman (1996) referred to the ABCs of addressing vicarious traumatization: awareness, balance, and connection. Every intervention strategy for vicarious traumatization is based upon mindfulness and acceptance (see Figure 3). Mindfulness is insight into the experience of vicarious traumatization, and acceptance must take

---

Figure 3. Vicarious Traumatization Intervention Strategies for Each Realm of the Nurse's Life

Personal
- Making personal life a priority
- Personal psychotherapy
- Leisure activities: physical, creative, spontaneous, relaxing
- Spiritual well-being
- Nurturing all aspects of the self: emotional, physical, spiritual, interpersonal, creative, artistic
- Attention to health

Professional
- Supervision and consultation
- Scheduling: patient load and distribution
- Balance and variety of tasks
- Education: giving and receiving
- Workspace

Organizational
- Collegial support
- Forums to address vicarious traumatization
- Supervision availability
- Respect for clinicians and patients
- Resources: mental health benefits, space, time

In All Realms
- Mindfulness and self-awareness
- Self-nurturance
- Balance: work, play, rest
- Meaning and connection

Note. From *Transforming the Pain: A Workbook on Vicarious Traumatization* (p. 85), by K.W. Saakvitne and L.A. Pearlman, 1996, New York, NY: W.W. Norton & Company. Copyright 1996 by the Traumatic Stress Institute/Center for Adult & Adolescent Psychotherapy LLC. Reprinted with permission.

REFLECTION

Making a Commitment to Yourself

Write down three things you could do to address vicarious traumatization for each realm of your life. Reflect upon the behaviors below and think about what changes you can make in the next week, next month, or next year. Focus on positive change.

Personal

_____
_____
_____
_____
_____

Professional

_____
_____
_____
_____
_____

Organizational

_____
_____
_____
_____
_____

Health

_____
_____
_____
_____
_____

Note. From *Transforming the Pain: A Workbook on Vicarious Traumatization* (p. 95), by K.W. Saakvitne and L.A. Pearlman, 1996, New York, NY: W.W. Norton & Company. Copyright 1996 by the Traumatic Stress Institute/Center for Adult & Adolescent Psychotherapy LLC. Reprinted with permission.

place before change or transformation. Until the nurse is willing to identify vulnerability to vicarious traumatization, prevention and positive change cannot happen.

Summary

The construct of vicarious traumatization can be differentiated from burnout and compassion fatigue. In vicarious traumatization, the nurse's inner belief system related to self and others becomes damaged. The nurse loses faith in life issues related to safety, trust, predictability, and protection. The inner experience or cognitive schema of the nurse changes in response to cumulative loss and suffering. A personal history of trauma increases the risk of vicarious traumatization. Behaviors that the nurse may exhibit include those associated with burnout and compassion fatigue but additionally include feelings of helplessness and impotency about "the system" and life in general (Blair & Ramones, 1996). The nurse experiencing unresolved vicarious traumatization is at high risk for symptoms of STSD, depression, and anxiety (see Chapters 4, 8, and 9). The goal is for the nurse to address the isolation and disillusionment associated with vicarious traumatization (Blair & Ramones, 1996) and work toward regaining a sense of self and personal and professional grounding.

Case Study

Sharon had worked on a hospice unit for more than two years and in the specialty of oncology for almost 20 years. When she began working in oncology, she had attended an in-depth certification course and was proud to be certified in her specialty. Sharon was passionate about her work and found reciprocal emotional rewards from her patients and their families. She had decided to specialize in hospice when her mother died of breast cancer at 65 years old. Hospice had been very supportive of her mother and the family during the terminal stage of disease. Sharon felt that she had never experienced such compassion and caring in her nursing career as that given during her mother's death. She felt inspired to be a caregiver like those role-modeled to her. She felt she had the insight, compassion, and empathy to be present for patients and families who, like her mother, needed comfort during the end of life.

The inpatient hospice experience was not living up to Sharon's expectations. Although it was a small unit, it was understaffed and always busy. The patients she cared for were terminally ill and in need of intense emotional support, day in and day out. Families also hovered over their loved ones, and Sharon cared for their emotional needs as well. But because of the limited resources and the organizational tasks that were required in her job, Sharon was unable to hold the hands of patients as she had envisioned. She always felt in a hurry, and even when she held the hand of a dying patient, Sharon had a million other things on her mind. There was no sense of balance between patient needs and work demands. Support was also minimal. Except for the unit director and the palliative care physician, there were not enough experienced and caring nurses to go around. The chaplain would make rounds, but neither he nor the psychologist on staff would ever ask staff members how they were doing.

Initially, Sharon didn't notice the subtle changes in herself. Normally a happy-go-lucky individual, she now found herself serious and somewhat pessimistic. At work she became cynical and always made negative remarks to colleagues regarding short-staffing and institutional protocols: "*Is this how the CEO would want his family members treated if they were on our unit?*" Resentment began to build as Sharon became emotionally and physically exhausted. She would be with a dying patient with breast cancer and have flashbacks about her own mother's early death. She began to feel angry about her own losses and those of the family members she would comfort when their loved one died. Her feelings peaked one day and she had an inappropriate interchange with the unit's director, demanding, "*How can you sleep at night knowing that we are not giving our patients the care they need and deserve?*" Actually, it was Sharon who was having trouble sleeping at night, and she felt she was not giving her patients enough of her attention to meet their needs. She stopped feeling sad or tearful and instead began to

Notes

feel angry at herself and others. "Life is not fair," she began think-ing. Sharon also began to fear that her stress level would eventual-ly contribute to the same fate that her mother confronted.

A few months later, Sharon noticed a change in every aspect of her life. Since she began working on the hospice unit, she had dropped her exercise routine as she found herself missing classes because of late nights at work. She could not muster the energy to attend her monthly specialty organization meetings, and her colleagues stopped going out after work together, which had initially been cus-tomary. She didn't have the energy to socialize with her friends out-side of work. She assumed that they would not want to listen to her feelings or care about her work issues. Sharon felt she had nowhere and no one to turn to. Her husband hated to hear about her work. His usual reply to any story she shared was, "That is so depressing."

Discussion

In this case, Sharon was showing definitive signs of vicarious traumatization. She showed signs of burnout: physical and emo-tional exhaustion. Organizational structure was contributing to Sharon's symptoms of vicarious traumatization. Short-staffing and limited resources in such a high-intensity patient population will contribute to nurses' feeling overwhelmed and overextend-ed with resultant feelings of decreased self-esteem and self-effica-cy. Sharon also displayed feelings of irritability, anxiety, and an-ger. The outburst projected onto her unit director was not nor-mally part of Sharon's character. She also started to withdraw and isolate herself from her normal social activities, and she felt there was no one she could trust, including her husband, with her deep-est feelings and emotions.

Sharon did not feel as though she could give enough of her-self to meet her patients' needs. She was also experiencing diffi-culty sleeping and flashbacks related to the unresolved grief over her mother's death. Sharon's positive hospice experience during her mother's death was a constant reminder of what her patients were *not* getting.

In this case, it would benefit Sharon to go into individual psy-chotherapy to work through her simmering personal and profes-sional grief. She has lost faith and trust in her normal support resources, so an objective counselor could benefit Sharon's need for her own emotional support and understanding. Counseling also could help Sharon learn how to set limits and to not feel that she was alone and the sole person responsible for meeting the needs of the patients on her unit. Sharon's feelings of safety and trust may return and allow her to experience the support of colleagues and supervisors. A counselor could role-play with Sharon and make suggestions on how she could approach her colleagues to help her when needed and to brainstorm about ways to bring the team together. With limited organizational resources, reaching out for help and teamwork is an important buffer against cumulative vicarious traumatization. Identifying how she can make positive changes across the personal, professional, and organizational aspects of her life will increase Sharon's sense of control.

With counseling, Sharon may not feel that her husband or friends have to be active listeners concerning her job. Instead, they could be social support for other activities necessary for Sharon's healing: fun, play, and laughter. Sharon also could suggest that the chaplain or the psychologist carry out bereavement meetings and also be available to individuals who may need brief grief counseling after a patient's death. She could carry out activities to help with her own grief, such as meditation, journaling, guided imagery, and other healing activities. If Sharon learns that self-care is necessary for her emotional rejuvenation and learns to set boundaries, then she may be able to delegate, leave her shift on time, and resume her exercise class. Finally, Sharon needs to identify what is *meaningful* to her in both her personal and professional life. Only activities that are meaningful and individualized for her will defuse her vicarious traumatization.

Notes

References

Blair, D.T., & Ramones, V.A. (1996). Understanding vicarious traumatization. *Journal of Psychosocial Nursing and Mental Health Services, 34*(11), 24–30.

Boelen, P.A., & Huntjens, R.J. (2008). Intrusive images in grief: An exploratory study. *Clinical Psychology and Psychotherapy, 15,* 217–226. doi:10.1002/cpp.568

Lavoie, S., Talbot, L.R., & Mathieu, L. (2011). Post-traumatic stress disorder symptoms among emergency nurses: Their perspective and a 'tailor-

Notes

made' solution. *Journal of Advanced Nursing, 67,* 1514–1522. doi:10.1111/j.1365-2648.2010.05584.x

Pearlman, L.A., & MacIan, P.S. (1995). Vicarious traumatization: An empirical study of the effects of trauma work on trauma therapists. *Professional Psychology: Research and Practice, 26,* 558–565.

Saakvitne, K.W., & Pearlman, L.A. (1996). *Transforming the pain: A workbook on vicarious traumatization.* New York, NY: W.W. Norton & Company.

Sinclair, H.A., & Hamill, C. (2007). Does vicarious traumatisation affect oncology nurses? A literature review. *European Journal of Oncology Nursing, 11,* 348–356. doi:10.1016/j.ejon.2007.02.007

Recommended Reading

Harrison, R.L., & Westwood, M.J. (2009). Preventing vicarious traumatization of mental health therapists: Identifying protective practices. *Psychotherapy, 46,* 203–219. doi:10.1037/a0016081

Laposa, J.M., Alden, L.E., & Fullerton, L.M. (2003). Work stress and posttraumatic stress disorder in ED nurses/personnel. *Journal of Emergency Nursing, 29,* 23–28. doi:10.1067/men.2003.7

McCann, I.L., & Pearlman, L.A. (1990). Vicarious traumatization: A framework for understanding the psychological effects of working with victims. *Journal of Traumatic Stress, 3,* 131–149. doi:10.1007/BF00975140

Rothschild, B. (with Rand, M.L.). (2006). *Help for the helper: The psychophysiology of compassion fatigue and vicarious trauma.* New York, NY: W.W. Norton & Company.

Internet Resources

Cavalcade Productions, Inc. Video Series on Vicarious Traumatization: www.cavalcadeproductions.com/vicarious-traumatization.html

Self-Care Academy: www.self-careacademy.com

Vicarious Trauma Institute: www.vicarioustrauma.com

SECONDARY TRAUMATIC STRESS DISORDER

Introduction

U nattended, prolonged stress and sorrow may leave the nurse vulnerable to the end of the burnout continuum, a concept termed *secondary traumatic stress disorder* (STSD). Also termed *traumatic stress reaction*, STSD refers to nurses being exposed to traumatic experiences of patients and vicariously taking in the emotional pain of those they care for. It is the conscious and unconscious actions, behaviors, or memories associated with experiences that are so traumatically stressful that they change the psychological resources available to the nurse and are severe enough to cause pathology (Figley, 1999). STSD is viewed as a construct similar to post-traumatic stress disorder, or PTSD (Stamm, 1999). Criteria related to PTSD are outlined in Figure 4. STSD results from a combination of the nurse's own previous traumatic experiences and the trauma experienced with patients. STSD also is related to the *empathic response* of the nurse to the patient (Dominguez-Gomez & Rutledge, 2009).

Empathy is the central force in what Wilson and Thomas (2004) termed *traumatoid states*—comprising compassion fatigue, vicarious traumatization, and STSD. *Empathy* is defined as connectedness between the nurse and patient, and the concept implies a positive and mutual relationship of trust, understanding, and a willingness to stay present in the healing pro-

Notes

Figure 4. Criteria for Post-Traumatic Stress Disorder
• **Criterion A:** The person has been exposed to a traumatic event and responds with intense fear, helplessness, or horror.
• **Criterion B:** The trauma is reexperienced through recurrent and distressing thoughts, dreams, or nightmares of the trauma.
• **Criterion C:** The person exhibits avoidance behaviors such as decreased interest in activities, feelings of detachment or estrangement from others, and restricted affect or emotional numbing.
• **Criterion D:** The person experiences persistent symptoms such as difficulty falling asleep or staying asleep, difficulty concentrating, irritability, or outbursts of anger.
• **Criterion E:** Criteria B, C, and D persist for more than one month.
• **Criterion F:** The disturbance causes clinically significant distress and interferes with social and occupational functioning and other activities.

Note. Based on information from American Psychiatric Association, 2000.

cess. It is the establishment of mutuality and trust. "Empathy embraces many of the highest qualities of human nature: compassion for others, authentic understanding and communication, openness to experience, respect for human dignity, and a willingness to reach out and help others in unselfish ways" (Wilson & Thomas, 2004, p. 143). Stebnicki (2008) grouped all the fatigue syndromes and labeled them as *empathy fatigue.* Professionals who use person-centered, empathy-focused interactions are seen as most susceptible to empathy fatigue. Research has shown that empathy appears to be both a personality trait and a state trait that most people possess. Professional caregivers such as nurses must be aware of when their empathic traits and states are being strained and exhausted. A mind-body connection appears to exist between empathy, an emotional and psychologically based experience, and physical fatigue, a physiologic condition of decreased functioning (Stebnicki, 2008).

If empathic caring is at the core of many fatigue syndromes, then it is not surprising that nurses who work in high-stress environments with intense patient populations are at greatest risk for STSD. Nurses become very resilient and demonstrate effective coping mechanisms, but prolonged exposure to stressors without personal or professional resources will contribute to stress-related symptoms. Symptoms of STSD are both physical and psychological and range from the fight-or-flight response to complete immobilization, similar to symptoms of anxiety (see Chapter 9). Stress symptoms are outlined in Table 1. Long-term effects of STSD include suppression of emotions, the reluctance to acknowledge trauma, concern regarding the perceptions of others, and distancing (Badger, 2001). In nurses suffering from STSD, a common behavioral response is to withdraw from others, avoid personal intimacy with patients, and eventually distance themselves from relationships outside of the workplace (see Table 1).

Personal coping skills influence the risk of STSD. Coping skills are enhanced by years of experience in nursing, educational preparation for the role, competency level, physical and mental health, and comparable situations previously experienced. Nurses who have experienced personal trauma (e.g., childhood trauma, emotional abuse, unresolved grief) are predisposed to STSD. Nurses in particular are susceptible to traumatic stress because of

Table 1. Stress Responses in Secondary Traumatic Stress Disorder

Symptom	Definition
Denial and shock	The nurse feels that everything is happening in slow motion.
Overwhelmed	The nurse becomes cognitively immobilized and does not know how to think or act.
Emotional numbing	The nurse becomes withdrawn, has a decreased capacity for pleasure, and demonstrates emotional instability, restlessness, or pessimism.
Acute stress disorder	The nurse experiences acute stress responses such as tachycardia and fight-or-flight responses.
Secondary traumatic stress disorder	Symptoms similar to those with post-traumatic stress disorder are present: hyperarousal, nightmares, and flashbacks.

Note. Based on information from Badger, 2001.

Notes

Notes

their perceived lack of control over traumatic incidents and congruent concern about professional competency in dealing with traumatic events (Badger, 2001). Nurses cope more effectively when they feel prepared, competent, and able to exert control during an event (Badger, 2001).

In the development of the Clinicians' Trauma Reaction Survey, Wilson and Thomas (2004) identified five factors that reflected therapists' reactions to trauma work. These factors can easily be applied to the work of nurses exposed to trauma over time. The factors are outlined in Figure 5. The factors identify the risk of empathic strain, which may lead to STSD.

- **Factor I.** STSD is indicative of the nurse reexperiencing the psychological distress of the patient. The nurse can become preoccupied with the unwanted thoughts or feelings of the trauma or stress that the patient is experiencing. The nurse can experience the same strong emotional reactions that the patient and family are demonstrating. Physiologic reactions of the nurse are similar to symptoms of PTSD that the patient may be experiencing. These include sleep disorders, nightmares, hypervigilance, and an exaggerated startle response. Inherent in this factor are symptoms of vicarious traumatization. The nurse may find a change in personal constructs such as worldview, self-identity, and systems of believing and meaning.

- **Factor II.** Defined as avoidance and detachment, reactions that include a loss of concentration, distraction, emotional numbing, and memory problems are involved in STSD. The detachment behaviors that can occur with STSD can be harmful to pa-

---

Figure 5. Five Factors Reflecting Empathic Strain

Factor I—Intrusive preoccupation with the nature of trauma work experiences

Factor II—Avoidance and detachment

Factor III—Overinvolvement and identification

Factor IV—Professional alienation

Factor V—Professional role satisfaction

Note. Based on information from Wilson & Thomas, 2004.

tient care. The nurse may avoid intimate conversations with the patient or become preoccupied with personal issues, thus not using listening skills that are inherent in quality patient care. Somatic complaints such as fatigue and headaches are also part of avoidance and detachment.

- **Factor III.** This factor is defined as overinvolvement and identification, the opposite of avoidance and detachment. These behaviors include overprotectiveness of the patient and feeling personally involved with the patient (for example, becoming the advocate or feeling like the liberator or patient's savior) (Wilson & Thomas, 2004). In these cases, the nurse may begin to behave with anger against life and society, actively viewing the world as unjust and unfair, similar to vicarious traumatization.

- **Factor IV.** This factor is defined as professional alienation. The nurse becomes distrustful of peers, colleagues, and supervisors, establishing feelings of isolation and behaviors of withdrawal. This factor also includes the nurse losing interest in normally enjoyable activities and losing a sense of sensuality and emotional sensitivity (Wilson & Thomas, 2004). As the nurse becomes emotionally "numb," mistrust and anxiety prevent the nurse from sharing with others the emotional impact and drain of the work. The danger here is that the nurse becomes further isolated in pain and fear, and self-disclosure becomes impossible.

- **Factor V.** Factor V is the opposite of alienation; it is professional role satisfaction. It is characterized by positive feelings toward work and working with challenging patient populations. Wilson and Thomas (2004) called this *empathic equilibrium,* a state in which helpers maintain clear boundaries, sustain a sense of professional meaning in their work, and have a sense of meaning in their life. This balance promotes positive transformation in both the patient and the nurse. Yet, inherent dangers in professional commitment include the inability to maintain balance in boundary setting, meeting one's own needs through work with patients, or making the job the only avenue for self-satisfaction and personal growth.

Notes

REFLECTION

Empathic Engagement

Review the five factors for risk of empathic strain and reflect upon your feelings and reactions to the following situations. Reply true or false. There are no wrong or right answers.

Factor I. Intrusive Preoccupation With the Nature of Trauma Work Experiences

_____ After working with my patients, I find myself always thinking about or "haunted" by what is happening to them.

_____ I find that I am reacting to situations the way that my patients might (e.g., on edge, anxious, irritable, exaggerated startle response).

_____ My work makes me worry more about the safety of those I hold dear.

_____ Because of the intensity of my work, I have found myself reappraising my own beliefs.

Factor II. Avoidance and Detachment

_____ While listening to my patients, I have noticed that my thoughts drift elsewhere.

_____ I find myself fatigued and drowsy while working with my patients.

_____ I feel myself "numbing out" while listening to my patients.

_____ I experience emotional detachment while working with my patients.

Factor III. Overinvolvement and Identification

_____ I experience protective feelings toward my patients.

_____ I have experienced a need to rescue, shelter, or save my patients.

_____ I am deeply touched by my patients and their stories and traumas.

_____ I have done more for my patients than is required by my professional role.

Factor IV. Professional Alienation

_____ I do not feel safe or trusting of my colleagues or supervisors to talk about my work or my concerns in working with challenging patients.

_____ Because of my work with patients, I feel alienated from others who do not understand the work that I do.

_____ I have felt abandoned by my colleagues and supervisors related to my work with patients.

_____ I find it difficult to share with others some of the horrific stories about my patients.

Factor V. Professional Role Satisfaction

_____ I find a heightened awareness of meaning for living or reason for being because of my work with patients.

_____ I find it difficult to maintain firm boundaries with my patients because of their needs.

_____ I have experienced feelings of not wanting to continue to work with specific patients because of the intensity of their care.

_____ Because of the nature of my work, I often wish that I were doing something different in my career.

Note. Based on information from Wilson & Thomas, 2004.

Interventions

The goals of treatment for nurses suffering from STSD are focused on functional improvement in job performance and reduction of the core disabling symptoms (Foa, Keane, & Friedman, 2000). Education regarding the causes and symptoms of STSD is the first step for nurses to gain insight into venues of self-healing. Understanding the interrelationships between burnout, compassion/empathy fatigue, and vicarious traumatization can prevent nurses from traveling the continuum to the stage of STSD. Continuous self-assessment of healthy lifestyle behaviors and effective coping strategies is essential for nurses who are working in high-stress environments or with high-intensity patient populations. Colleagues and supervisors also can help nurses recognize harmful emotional responses (such as blurred boundaries) or harmful behaviors (such as outbursts of anger). A safe and trusting work environment is another essential ingredient for prevention of STSD for individual nurses and for the entire staff working as a team.

High-risk symptoms that necessitate intervention include the danger of harming oneself or others, the inability to carry out normal life activities, or the need for psychiatric evaluation if the individual is struggling with major psychological issues, such as prolonged grief, depression, or anxiety (see Chapters 5, 8, and 9). "The greater the demand and/or the fewer the resources the person has with which to make the change, the greater the potential for the stress to be traumatic or even pathological" (Stamm, 1999, p. xxxviii). Symptoms of STSD are congruent to those of patients with PTSD, and interventions are similar. Stages of treatment are outlined in Figure 6. *Ensuring safety is the number-one priority.* Psychological support may be in the form of support groups or individual psychotherapy if needed. Cognitive-behavioral therapy, art and music therapy, relaxation techniques, and guided imagery are all healing interventions. Under the guidance of a psychiatrist, the use of psychopharmacology may be effective in the treatment of sleep disorders, anxiety, depression, and acute stress disorder. As with the majority of psychiatric disorders, a combination of treatment strategies individualized toward targeting the

Notes

Figure 6. Components of Treatment for Secondary Traumatic Stress Disorder

- Ensure safety.
- Create a safe and secure environment.
- Aim for stabilization—symptom containment and reduction.
- Emphasize grounding—being in the here and now.
- Allow remembrance and mourning, both personal and professional.
- Encourage nurses to talk about their trauma. Be sensitive in inquiring about grief and loss.
- Be emotionally supportive; meet nurses where they are at the present time.
- Create choices for management and control.
- Reassure nurses that it is common to experience distressing symptoms while reinforcing effective coping skills, progress, and mastery in managing symptoms.
- Relieve irrational guilt.
- Provide education about acute stress and post-traumatic stress responses.
- Normalize the experience as a biologic reaction that causes changes in the brain (which helps to find ways to cope).
- Aim to restructure traumatic/personal schemas.
- Aim to reestablish secure social connections and interpersonal efficacy.
- Repair emotional experiences.
- Rebuild self-esteem, self-confidence, and self-efficacy in all major life activities.

Note. Based on information from Johnson, 2009.

---

nurse's most pressing symptoms may prove the most promising (Bush, 2009).

Again, supportive interventions also are needed within the work environment. Treatment should be multidisciplinary with a team approach using the resources of advanced practice nurses (APNs), nurse managers, staff therapists, and pastoral services. Routine support groups should be focused on ways to improve effective coping resources at the individual level and effective teamwork at the staff level. An honest, open, and trusting environment will allow nurses to feel safe to express emotions of hurt, frustration, fear, and anxiety. Normalizing these feelings is important for nurses to understand that they are not isolated in these responses. Often, role-playing or using case studies aids the team in understanding effective emotional and behavioral responses to difficult patients and situations. Stamm (1999) referred to normalizing stress as the "self-changing nature of caregiving" (p. xxxviii). Education includes teaching nurses about not only the emotional and psychological responses to stress but also the somatic responses, for example, fight-or-flight reaction in acute anxiety. Interventions to manage somatic experiences may include education regarding relaxation techniques, deep breathing, and imagery. Teaching nurses how to self-monitor arousal states and ways to control or effectively manage their responses can prevent feelings of uncontrolled anxiety (see Chapter 9).

Summary

STSD is the presence of PTSD symptoms in the caregiver. This results from a combination of the caregiver's own traumatic history and the trauma experiences of the caregiver's patients (Dominguez-Gomez & Rutledge, 2009). STSD is closely related to and is on the continuum of burnout, compassion fatigue, and vicarious traumatization. The experience of STSD is cumulative and related to prolonged exposure to suffering and traumatized patients. Symptoms of STSD involve reexperiencing the trauma of the patient, avoiding stimuli associated with the trauma, and experiencing symptoms of increased arousal. Dealing with organizational and personal stressors and seeking resources such as psychotherapy are important for the nurse to resolve STSD.

Case Study

Joyce was a second-year graduate student specializing in pediatrics. She worked the night shift in the pediatric critical care unit at a tertiary care referral center an hour away from her home. Joyce was in her early 40s and had gotten remarried the previous

Notes

summer. She shared custody of her elementary school–aged children with her previous husband. Her new spouse, a physician, was supportive of her children and her professional work and graduate studies. Joyce's husband was also very busy in his own private cardiology practice. However, he did not put demands on Joyce's time when she needed to juggle all of her activities with the children, work, and school. Joyce also had support from her younger sister and teenage nieces who lived close by and often helped her with child care.

Joyce had worked in pediatrics for almost 20 years. She decided to go back to school because she found herself weary and bored with her staff nurse role. Joyce felt that she could not do enough for her patients and that she had little control over what happened on the unit, especially because she worked the night shift. She hoped that becoming a clinical nurse specialist (CNS) would guarantee her a job in pediatric critical care and more control over what she believed could be done for patients, their families, and fellow staff members.

Joyce was not prepared for the rigors of school. Additionally, even though her husband was supportive, her recent marriage came with new emotional and social demands. Her husband frequently worked very late hours and did not seem available when Joyce needed him. Her 12-hour shifts sometimes became 13-plus hours with only a brief break for a quick bite to eat. In recent years, the staff had been asked to do more with fewer and fewer resources, including staffing. The night shift was as busy as the day shift and frequently even more demanding. Families were not always available to help patients, and ancillary staff presence was marginal at best. The children became fearful at night with fears and fantasies abounding. Joyce often wanted to stop and stay with them for a few extra moments to provide comfort, but this was rarely an option of late. There never seemed to be enough time. Joyce frequently complained to her nurse manager that more support staff was needed during the night shift, but this lament seemed to fall on deaf ears. Now after what seemed like years of complaining, she just felt resentful and angry, especially toward her peers on the day shift, who she didn't think understood what it was like to work nights. At times, Joyce felt as though the night shift employees were treated as second-class citizens.

Recently, Joyce had found herself often thinking about her patients during daytime hours when she should have been sleeping or caring for her children. She worried about her patients' welfare when she wasn't caring for them personally. Joyce feared that a special long-term patient, a preschooler she had grown fond of, would die when she wasn't working. She found herself identifying with and thinking more about the parents of her patients. It became harder and harder for Joyce to focus on her studies. At times she felt hopeless that she would ever achieve her long-term goal of becoming a CNS, and if she did, would it even make a difference? When she tried to talk to her husband about her professional concerns, he couldn't really understand the pressure and stress she felt. His responses seemed conciliatory: "You always complain about your work, but you are going to school because you want to, not because you have to." Soon Joyce found herself not expecting much support from her husband, her peers, or her nurse manager. She started keeping her feelings to herself. She felt almost numb, going from one expectation to another, feeling fragmented and disconnected from everything and everyone. Her anxiety began to build. Joyce felt increasingly nervous and irritable along with experiencing unsettling feelings of doom. She felt as though she was constantly nagging her husband and children and wasn't enjoying her time with them. Joyce also regretted not having time to spend with her sister or friends, but then she didn't feel they could support her or understand her anyway.

Discussion

Joyce is demonstrating symptoms of STSD. She appears to feel overwhelmed in all aspects of her life—cognitively immobilized and unable to feel, think, or act appropriately. Although Joyce's husband saw her as calm and confident, inwardly Joyce felt the opposite: anxious and incompetent. She worried that she was unable to perform her best at school or at work with her patients. She became irritable with her children and found less and less enjoyment in spending time with them because of the

Notes

pressure to study. She was withdrawing from her peers at work and not disclosing her emotional feelings of stress with anyone. Joyce felt abandoned and alienated; no one would understand how she felt if she even tried to explain, she thought. She found herself feeling emotionally numb and unable to be attentive in caring for or listening to her patients. This proved very disconcerting, as she had been very empathetic and an excellent listener.

Joyce would benefit from both individual psychotherapy and from a more secure and safe work environment. Cognitive-behavioral therapy could help Joyce to reframe the negative thoughts that were damaging her feelings of self-esteem and self-efficacy. In the safety of therapy, Joyce could learn to trust again and gain insight into her own behaviors of isolation and withdrawal. A therapist could also diagnose any significant psychological problems affecting Joyce, such as acute stress disorder or depression. Cognitive-behavioral therapy could help Joyce to identify how she could support and care for her patients while setting firm boundaries between her work obligations and her personal life.

Pediatric critical care is a challenging specialty. It involves intense emotional caring and high-level mastery of the physiologic sequelae of life-threatening illness in the most valued cohort of society—young children. The organizational environment must become sensitive to workplace stressors and provide ancillary support to staff practicing on both day and night shifts. As Joyce receives help in individual therapy, she also could learn how to reach out and express her emotional needs in a more positive manner. She could find an effective approach to discuss the special night shift needs with her manager and brainstorm some effective strategies to help these colleagues. In Joyce's case study, it is evident how the feelings and behaviors of one individual reverberate through professional and personal relationships. Inversely, Joyce's peers made no attempts to reach out to her to offer help. At home, her husband was unable to respond to her anxiety because Joyce was suppressing her true feelings and fears. Relationships are interdependent in nature. If this downward-spiraling domino effect of distress could be countered, then Joyce, her family, and her patients would benefit.

References

American Psychiatric Association. (2000). *Diagnostic and statistical manual of mental disorders* (4th ed., text rev.). Washington, DC: Author.

Badger, J.M. (2001). Understanding secondary traumatic stress. *American Journal of Nursing, 101*(7), 26–32.

Bush, N.J. (2009). Post-traumatic stress disorder related to the cancer experience. *Oncology Nursing Forum, 36*, 395–400. doi:10.1188/09.ONF .395-400

Dominguez-Gomez, E., & Rutledge, D.N. (2009). Prevalence of secondary traumatic stress among emergency nurses. *Journal of Emergency Nursing, 35*, 199–204. doi:10.1016/j.jen.2008.05.003

Figley, C. (1999). Compassion fatigue: Toward a new understanding of the costs of caring. In B.H. Stamm (Ed.), *Secondary traumatic stress: Self-care issues for clinicians, researchers, and educators* (2nd ed., pp. 3–28). Lutherville, MD: Sidran Press.

Foa, E.B., Keane, T.M., & Friedman, M.J. (2000). Guidelines for treatment of PTSD. *Journal of Traumatic Stress, 13*, 539–588. doi:10.1023/ A:1007802031411

Johnson, S.L. (2009). *Therapist's guide to posttraumatic stress disorder intervention.* San Diego, CA: Academic Press.

Stamm, B.H. (1999). Introduction to the first edition. In B.H. Stamm (Ed.), *Secondary traumatic stress: Self-care issues for clinicians, researchers, and educators* (2nd ed., pp. xxxiii–xliii). Lutherville, MD: Sidran Press.

Stebnicki, M.A. (2008). *Empathy fatigue: Healing the mind, body, and spirit of professional counselors.* New York, NY: Springer.

Wilson, J.P., & Thomas, R.B. (2004). *Empathy in the treatment of trauma and PTSD.* New York, NY: Brunner-Routledge.

Recommended Reading

Beck, C.T. (2011). Secondary traumatic stress in nurses: A systematic review. *Archives of Psychiatric Nursing, 25*, 1–10. doi:10.1016/j.apnu.2010.05.005

Levine, S. (2005). *Unattended sorrow: Recovering from loss and reviving the heart.* Emmaus, PA: Rodale.

Meadors, P., & Lamson, A. (2008). Compassion fatigue and secondary traumatization: Provider self care on intensive care units for children. *Journal of Pediatric Health Care, 22*, 24–34. doi:10.1016/j.pedhc.2007.01 .006

Meadors, P., Lamson, A., Swanson, M., White, M., & Sira, N. (2009–2010). Secondary traumatization in pediatric healthcare providers: Compassion fatigue, burnout, and secondary traumatic stress. *Omega, 60*, 103–128.

Mealer, M., Burnham, E.L., Goode, C.J., Rothbaum, B., & Moss, M. (2009). The prevalence and impact of post traumatic stress disorder and burnout syndrome in nurses. *Depression and Anxiety, 26*, 1118–1126. doi:10.1002/ da.20631

Notes

Notes

Quinal, L., Harford, S., & Rutledge, D.N. (2009). Secondary traumatic stress in oncology staff. *Cancer Nursing, 32*(4), E1–E7. doi:10.1097/NCC.0b013e31819ca65a

Rothschild, B. (with Rand, M.L.). (2006). *Help for the helper: The psychophysiology of compassion fatigue and vicarious trauma.* New York, NY: W.W. Norton & Company.

Internet Resources

Beth Hudnall Stamm and Professional Quality of Life Scale: www.isu.edu/~bhstamm

Figley Institute: www.figleyinstitute.com/reading_room.html

Self-Care Academy: www.self-careacademy.com

NURSE GRIEF

Introduction

Grief is the emotional response (often referred to as *suffering*) to personal feelings of loss. It is the reaction to the absence of someone or something in which the griever was heavily invested. Grief can be conceptualized as stages, points in time, tasks, or themes, all focusing on the way individuals process, reconcile, and integrate loss into their life. Frequently referred to as a journey, grief is not a linear process characterized by a stepwise progression of feelings and responses. Rather, it is a complex, fluid, overlapping, changing series of distressing feelings and behaviors that evolve in prominence and intensity over time. Influenced by a host of factors, grief usually indicates some degree of mental suffering. In response to the death of a loved one, grief is commonly referred to as "having a broken heart."

Societal norms dictate how grieving individuals should act and respond. When expectations are not conformed to, negative judgment often is imposed such that the grieving person is perceived as somehow flawed in his or her response. The American standard exhorts stoicism and emotional concealment. Generally, expressions of sadness and remorse are not encouraged, except in supportive milieus. Statements that may prompt emotional triggers of grief reactions are avoided. Hence, many grievers report feeling alienated and isolated in their emotional pain. They remain acutely aware of how uncomfortable their loss makes those around them feel.

Notes

Recognition of the importance of grief work within health care evolved in tandem with the evolution of the death and dying movement within American culture. Figure 7 outlines a depiction of five grief models. These representations are efforts to categorize phases of grief. However, they are based primarily on anecdotal impressions and observations. Rigorous research is lacking to substantiate the many facets of grief (Konigsberg, 2011). Despite four decades of increasing attention and discourse, "normal" grief remains an anomaly.

Conventional wisdom about the pathology of grief has been challenged. Recent reports have confirmed that the majority who grieve the loss of a loved one do not suffer disabling symptoms that impair their ability to function, both acutely and long term (Bonanno, 2009). Only about 15% of people experience what is now termed *prolonged grief disorder*, a newly proposed psychiatric diagnosis reflective of a protracted, problem-ridden grief recovery trajectory (Bauer & Bonanno, 2001; Bonanno & Kaltman, 2001; Holland, Neimeyer, Boelen, & Prigerson, 2009). Personal characteristics of resilience, perseverance, and hardiness appear to be critical in offsetting the deleterious ramifications of grief. Hence, acknowledging the myriad controversies and quandaries surrounding the contemporary understanding of grief, it is not surprising that, like many of the phenomena addressed in this book, little is known about nurse grief.

Figure 7. Models of Grief Responses

Model 1	Model 2	Model 3	Model 4	Model 5
• Shock	• Numbness	• Recognize death	• Crisis	• Accepting the reality of loss
• Denial	• Yearning and searching	• React emotionally	• Unity	• Experiencing the pain of grief
• Anger	• Disorganization, anger, despair	• Recollect and reexperience	• Upheaval	• Adjusting to the environment in which the deceased is missing
• Bargaining	• Reorganization	• Relinquish	• Resolution	• Withdrawing emotional energy and investing in another relationship
• Acceptance		• Readjust	• Renewal	
		• Reinvest		

Note. Based on information from Konigsberg, 2011; Okun & Nowinski, 2011.

Grief experienced by nurses can be linked to two prominent antecedents (Boyle, 2006). First is the close, often intimate proximity that nurses have to patients over time. Nursing is emotional work that involves sharing an intimacy with the highly vulnerable. Second is the professional expectation to render compassionate care. Nursing care is substandard if it focuses on the physical to the exclusion of the humanistic component. This professionally imposed positioning and the expected emotive connectivity place nurses in circumstances of vulnerability. In particular, the phenomenon of empathic engagement can be a double-edged sword. On the positive side, it enhances the interpersonal connection with patients and families, thereby promoting their sense of being known and cared for. On the negative side, empathic engagement may be the source of profound sadness, even despondency, in nurses.

Exposure to loss in the work setting may be considerable for nurses. They observe patients lose their health, body parts, functional independence, roles, dignity, self-esteem, and their lives. Depending on the practice setting, nurses experience the death of their patients to acute or chronic illness, accidents, and other tragedies in both anticipated and unexpected time frames. In caring for critically ill and dying patients and their relatives, nurses must intervene in the most emotionally chaotic time of a family's life. They witness firsthand the dual losses that families endure, namely their identities (such as wife, son, or treasured grandchild) and their loved ones. Additionally, this close proximity of nurses to the dying experience often prompts a confrontation with their own mortality, which may heighten levels of anxiety and stress (Sherman, 2004).

Despite a growing recognition of the need to render holistic quality care to critically ill and dying patients, deterrents to such care prevail within the work setting. Many nurses feel ill-equipped to provide both highly sophisticated physical care and skilled therapeutic communication, and rarely is nurses' self-care addressed as a requisite competency within clinical practice (Boyle, 2011).

The denial of or the inability to cope with one's work-related grief may affect the nursing care provided to patients and families. Nurses may distance themselves from or not actively engage with patients and families, resulting in the absence of a therapeutic presence. With this exclusive focus on the practical, physical

Notes

needs of the patient, an avenue of escape evolves for the nurse. Emotionally charged topics can be avoided. Remaining "professional," a lauded ideal for some, requires compartmentalization of loss and sadness and the creation of a protective shell to mitigate grief. These reactions may negatively affect patient satisfaction. Workplace-derived grief that is avoided and unmanaged also may contribute to compassion fatigue (see Chapter 2). As a result, nurses may leave their position to work in an area or a role with less exposure to loss and death.

Nurses frequently provide compassionate care to the critically ill, dying, and bereaved with little attention given to their own emotions. Minimizing the emotional wear and tear on their own coping reserves devalues the critical nature of caring, a hallmark of nursing practice. Nurse grief work, if any, often involves discussions, usually superficial or informal in nature, with colleagues or friends. "Bottling it up" or crying alone (in the bathroom or during the car ride home) is common. Coworkers may listen to the nurse's sadness once a conversation is initiated. However, few colleagues systematically inquire about how their grieving nurse peers are faring. Support groups are infrequently offered, and the presence of on-site counselors is a rarity, particularly in ambulatory settings. A paucity of education is provided to nurses about the grief process. What usually is available relates to nursing interventions to support the grieving family, not how to take care of one's grieving self.

Numerous variables influence the nurse's grief response. Kearney, Weininger, Vachon, Harrison, and Mount (2011) identified common stressors for palliative care physicians that could influence grief, and these factors also have relevance for both the presence and intensity of nurse grief. These determinants include

- A growing caseload
- Constant exposure to death
- Inadequate time to spend with dying patients
- Disregard of personal emotional responses
- Need to "carry on as usual" in the wake of patients' deaths
- Communication difficulties with patients and families
- Developing friendships with patients and families
- Inability to live up to own standards
- Feelings of depression and guilt in response to loss.

REFLECTION

Acknowledging these common corollaries of contemporary health care, what scenarios or patient situations have made you cry or be on the brink of tears within the past six months? What situations do you continue to feel bad about or feel regret over? These may be indicative of unresolved grief.

_____

_____

_____

_____

_____

_____

_____

REFLECTION

Think of an individual patient who has died or a family member that you still occasionally think about. Once you have that image or name in mind, consider which of the following characteristics have meaning for this scenario.

• How well you knew the patient and family

• Your identification with the patient or family

• Nature of the disclosure of the prognosis or death

• Degree of team communication and interaction before and after the death

• Your presence at the time of death

• Your facilitation of family presence or post-death care

Your answers to these queries can help to identify risk factors related to your work-related grief responses. Do long-standing relationships that end with the patient's death prompt feelings of remorse? How does the degree of openness, secrecy, and honesty surrounding communication influence your reactions? Is it important that you be present at the time of death when a patient you deem "special" dies? Does your track record with facilitating family coping have an impact on your reaction? What is it about certain patients and families that fosters the creation of a special bond with them?

_____

_____

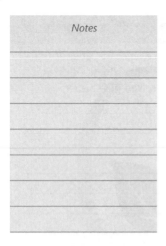

Notes

A critical variable to the understanding of nurse grief is the nature of the nurse-patient relationship (Lobb et al., 2010). Why do some patients become "special," warranting going the extra mile or remaining in the nurse's thoughts after work? A special bond may evolve when patients remind nurses of someone special in their lives (Sherman, 2004). Nurses may identify with those who are similar in age or life circumstances (Keidel, 2002). When nurses become close friends with patients, when they render care over and above the usual nursing care, the resultant grief engendered may be significantly increased. Personal pain can be exacerbated or guilt enhanced when these relationships end with the patient's death.

REFLECTION

The Empty Chair Dialogue

Think of a patient who has died and whom you still think about periodically. This patient should exemplify a loss to you because he or she was special. The goal of this reflection is to release feelings of sadness toward a particular patient in a safe way.

Directions: This exercise can be done alone or in a group. If you are completing this exercise as part of a group, place two chairs facing each other in the middle of a circle. Position the remaining chairs around you. Ask others in the group to listen to the dialogue and to consider giving their feedback at the completion of the exercise.

Sit in one chair and speak toward the empty chair facing you. Close your eyes and take some deep, soothing breaths, imagining the patient sitting across from you. Picture how the patient looks, what he or she is wearing, and the person's posture and facial expression. When you are ready, introduce the person you are speaking to, saying the patient's first name, the context in which you met, and when this contact occurred. Then verbally respond to the following four statements.
- You were a special patient to me because . . .
- What made me feel the saddest about your dying was . . .
- I wish I had . . .
- You taught me . . .

Now open up the discussion to all members of the group, asking them to share their reactions and impressions of the dialogue. What were the most compelling aspects of the exchange? What did you learn about yourself in hearing others' responses? In these cases demonstrating enduring memories involving a special patient who has died, a significant dose of "self-empathy" often is in order, as the death has highly personal implications beyond that usually experienced.

Note. Based on information from Field & Horowitz, 1998.

The intensity of time that nurses spend with patients and families often makes interpersonal connections highly significant. No other health professional claims the volume of time spent, the intimacy of the encounter, or the overall advocacy responsibilities associated with the coordination of patient care as nurses do. Nurses also may be confronted with waves of deaths and tragedy that at times overwhelm them with grief. The protracted nature of death exposure in highly tenured nurses deserves reflection.

Notes

REFLECTION

Cumulative Grief Inventory

This exercise requires paper and pencil. Its goal is twofold: to quantify the degree of loss and sadness you have experienced over your nursing career and to increase awareness of the scope of your cumulative grief. Calculate the following.

- Write down how many years you have been a nurse. _____

- Approximate how many dying patients and/or patients who actually died that you provided care to monthly (___); now multiply that number by 12 (___); then multiply that number by your total work years. TOTAL = _____

- Consider the number of deaths you have witnessed. Ask yourself, how many of these deaths have you grieved?

Special Note

Additionally, you may consider other stressful situations related to the dying experience. These may include caring for people who have attempted suicide, the number of codes and rapid responses you have participated in, how many times you have been in a patient's room just after the patient was given bad news or a dismal prognosis, how many stillborn deliveries or terminal weanings you have participated in, or the number of family-consoling interventions you have rendered.

Although the sum of one's grief is an important consideration, equally meaningful is the attention given to its resolution. When grief is not tended to, the by-products of loss-related sadness often accumulate, interfering with grief recovery. Terms such as *unresolved, complicated, pathologic,* or *prolonged* grief are labels affixed to this occurrence. These grief corollaries are thought to evolve when emotional avoidance is the preferred coping strategy and unattended sorrow is the norm.

Notes

Compounding the intensity of grief responses is the frequently blurred boundary between work and home. While the deaths of loved ones in the nurse's personal life are highly influential, so are numerous other sources of loss and sadness that influence the rendering of compassionate nursing care. These include, for example, marital separation or divorce, children leaving home, assuming a new job, or undertaking a geographical move. A sense of considerable emotional depletion may prevail when grief emanates from both home and work, especially if the losses remain unaddressed and unresolved.

REFLECTION

Loss Inventory

The goal of this exercise is to highlight the degree of personal loss in your life that may influence your nursing practice. In the following table, write down all of your losses within the appropriate time frame. Losses may include people or may involve illness, children, moving, or job changes. Highlight with a marker the time frames where significant loss was evident.

Age Span	Losses	Your Reaction
0–5		
6–10		
11–15		
16–20		
21–25		
26–30		
31–35		
36–40		

(Continued on next page)

REFLECTION *(CONTINUED)*		
Age Span	**Losses**	**Your Reaction**
41–45		
46–50		
51–55		
56–60		
61–65		
66 and older		

Now reflect on your current age and note what has transpired recently and in the more distant past. Are you surprised with the depiction of your losses? How did you cope with the sadness associated with these losses? What remains unresolved or complicated?

Interventions

As with all problem solving, solutions must be tailored to the nature of the event. Two major themes exist to consider in ameliorating the difficulties and demands associated with nurse grief: workplace implications and personal indices.

Within nursing, there often is a perception of weakness or self-indulgence when one acknowledges the need for help. This perception should be reframed. Articulating or naming the nature of distress promotes self-care and fosters intervention planning. Some recommendations for facilitating grief work for nurses include the following.

- Regularly scheduled group meetings with a psychiatric liaison clinical nurse specialist or counselor; these meetings should be promoted as forums to discuss common work setting scenarios that could benefit from open dialogue.
- One-on-one sessions with an available therapist

REFLECTION

Grief-Specific Questions to Consider in the Work Setting

Answer the following questions specific to your current work environment. Small focus group discussions are the ideal forum for this exchange.

How do I/we deal with grief following the death of a patient? _____

_____

_____

_____

Do we offer support to each other? _____

_____

_____

_____

How does our manager help us with our grief? _____

_____

_____

_____

Would more education about grief be helpful? _____

_____

_____

_____

What type of additional support (i.e., resources) could I/we benefit from? _____

_____

_____

_____

What are some "best practices" that could be incorporated into the work setting? _____

_____

_____

- Self-awareness training regarding death anxiety, dying, and grief
- Educational needs assessment related to aspects of end-of-life care that the nursing staff would like more skill building in
- End-of-life nursing care protocols that invite family participation in nursing care
- Debriefing sessions following a patient death to provide a review of the end-of-life process and to address staff grief reactions
- Bereavement programs in which cards are sent or telephone calls are made to families following the death of a loved one

All of these possibilities share common themes: enhanced communication, development of new skills, and promoting nurse mastery of end-of-life care.

Unique "best practices" also should be considered for replication. At City of Hope in Duarte, California, the "Tea for the Soul" intervention is facilitated by chaplains and pastoral care colleagues who render on-site support of nursing staff and address their emotional needs at the point of care (Di Rado, 2009). These regular events provide the nurses with time and encouragement to share stories with the chaplains and each other, relax, and enjoy refreshments, massages, and soothing music. The Department of Nursing at Roswell Park Cancer Institute in Buffalo, New York, has implemented a "Code Gray" program where a peer-based support intervention is offered to the nurse caring for a patient who just died ("Code Gray: Care for the Caregivers," 2008). The charge nurse or nurse manager facilitates a break time after a patient's death during which the staff nurse is encouraged to talk about the experience and, if needed, spend some time off the unit, such as visiting the hospital chapel.

Efforts to actively address the family's grief may in turn accommodate nurses' own grief responses. Novel offerings such as the creation of "grieving carts" for families maintaining vigils by the dying patient's bedside is a measure of highly compassionate caregiving. An intensive care unit at Banner Good Samaritan Medical Center in Phoenix, Arizona, created these carts to support families with the patient at the end of life. The unit

Notes

staff uses the cart to serve food and beverages to the family at the bedside, and a variety of religious materials and pamphlets are stored in the cart as well (Whitmer, Hurst, Stadler, & Ide, 2007). With an unexpected death such as a code, consideration should be given as to how the family views their loved one that promotes awareness of the healthcare team's efforts to save the patient (i.e., not cleaning and sterilizing the environment immediately after the death, leaving some equipment and materials from the code effort). Partnering with families in rituals that may facilitate their grief, such as helping with the final preparation of the body, taking a lock of the patient's hair, or creating memory boxes (often routinely done in hospice settings), may validate nurses' effectiveness in supporting grieving families. Although it is anecdotal in nature, some nurses find mutual benefit (for themselves and families) in participating in rituals such as funeral attendance to facilitate grief.

Paramount to improving nurse coping is offering training in areas often left to nurses to cultivate on their own. Of special note is communication skills training, a requisite competency in highly effective nursing care. Outside of the specialty of mental health nursing, nurses rarely receive instruction on how to speak with and counsel patients in crisis. Developing *exquisite empathy,* a contemporary term linked with the effective work of mental health therapists, has considerable applicability to nurses' sense of mastery in the provision of emotional support. Harrison and Westwood (2009) elucidated:

> "Exquisite empathy" requires a sophisticated balance on the part of the clinician as [he or she] simultaneously maintains clear and consistent boundaries, expanded perspective, and highly present, intimate, and heartfelt interpersonal connection in the therapeutic relationship . . . without fusing or losing sight of the clinician's own perspective. (p. 214)

Thus, it is that combination of connectedness in tandem with astute self-awareness that fosters the recognition of both possibilities and limitations within the patient encounter. This skill is highly relevant in the grief work of nurses.

REFLECTION

Nurse grief may become complicated for several reasons. You may experience ambiguous loss when a patient dies before you have the opportunity to say good-bye and have formal closure. You may in some measure feel responsible for a patient's death or may think you should have intervened on the patient's behalf differently or advocated more strongly for an intervention. In these cases, rational approximation of the your power to change a course of terminal events is required. Self-forgiveness may be in order. Consider a patient scenario from your past caseload where these feelings existed. Is your response guilt-ridden, and is it rational? Could you alone have changed the course of the patient's trajectory? Talk about your feelings within a supportive environment and ask for feedback from peers. Look within and also consider how your need to grieve parallels the depth of your attachment and involvement with the patient. Of utmost importance is your reflection of what you did or how you intervened to make the situation better. Describe your thoughts below.

An important approach to countering the negative effects of loss and grief is to purposefully reflect on the rewards gained from close interpersonal encounters with patients. Some examples of these include

- Appreciation for the reciprocal healing process, the lessons learned from the patient and family encounter (also labeled *vicarious post-traumatic growth*)
- Opportunity for inner self-reflection
- An enhanced sense of job engagement, a connection with peers and team members
- A heightened sense of spirituality
- Feelings of compassion satisfaction.

REFLECTION

Think of patients you have cared for over the past three months. In the following table, write the initials of three patients (or family members) in the left column that you remember most vividly. In the middle column, briefly describe what you did to ease their distress (i.e., physical, emotional, social, spiritual). What interventions did you employ to minimize their discomfort (for example, lobby for a medication change; touch, hold, or embrace them; engage in a conversation; request a consultation; provide information)? Consider how these individuals benefited from your orchestration of their care (i.e., end results).

Initials	Your Interventions	End Results

Embracing this reward orientation in the conceptualization of nursing outcomes may be an effective strategy used by highly tenured nurses who work in grief-laden nursing specialties. Sumner and Townsend-Rocchiccioli (2003) stated, "Even if its toll is recognized, it seems that the emotional human-to-human connection is what makes practice feasible" (p. 165).

Efforts to optimize self-awareness may include specific, targeted inventories (such as the reflective exercises described in this chapter) that promote an inner understanding of emotional responses and attachments. Journaling, a form of self-care, may foster personal awareness and self-understanding through reflection and emotive expression. *Mindfulness meditation* is a practice employed by clinicians to raise consciousness of their inner reactions and the external reality of how they are responding. Psychological benefits have been noted to include anxiety reduction, enhanced empathy, and a greater sense of self-directedness (Beddoe & Murphy, 2004; Kearney et al., 2011). These approaches offer a means to "calibrate" well-being by cultivating personal awareness.

Summary

Grief is a common yet somewhat controversial phenomenon in our culture. This chapter described key components of the underrecognized and understudied phenomenon of nurse grief. The reflective exercises provided will help to promote self-awareness and strategic planning specific to nurse grief. An enhanced understanding of outcomes related to highly emotive nurse work is necessary for the retention of a highly capable nursing workforce that provides holistic patient care. Personal and workplace interventions are necessary, as grief work requires purposeful attention in its successful navigation.

Case Study

Upon graduating from nursing school, Mary took a job in obstetrics within a teaching hospital that offered a special residency program for new graduates. She had previously worked as a nursing assistant in a float capacity and knew that labor and delivery was where she ultimately wanted to practice. Mary worked in the postpartum area for two years. She then got married and moved to southern California, where her husband was offered a job. Mary found a job at a large metropolitan hospital that had a growing perinatal high-risk program.

Mary soon became highly engaged in her unit. She chaired the unit's shared governance council. She led initiatives to develop support programs for the long-term mothers requiring lengthy hospitalizations. Many of the patients were similar in age to Mary. Families frequently wrote letters to the nurse manager about the exceptional, compassionate care Mary rendered. She was noted to frequently go above and beyond, visiting mothers and their babies after delivery. Mary was asked to teach and mentor the labor and delivery nurses about the unique aspects of the high-risk perinatal experience, focusing on early recognition of potential sequelae to reduce the likelihood of maternal morbidity and perinatal fatality.

One year after their move, Mary and her husband decided to start a family. She suffered two miscarriages before finally giving

Notes

birth to a healthy daughter. When her child was nine months old, Mary received a telephone call from her mother in the Midwest telling her that she had just been diagnosed with Alzheimer disease. Mary, an only child, was devastated. Baby in tow, she immediately went to visit her mother. Upon her arrival, Mary quickly realized that her mother was severely compromised. She was very confused, unable to care for herself, and was a considerable safety risk. Mary requested a family leave to care for her mother with the help of hospice home care. Within six weeks of Mary's visit, her mother died with Mary present.

Mary returned home, went back to work, and found herself feeling increasingly alienated from her patients. She still provided excellent nursing care, but she did not go the extra mile as she had before. Mary stopped her practice of visiting the mothers whom she had cared for and making telephone calls to families following the death of their preterm babies. Several months later, she became pregnant with her second child and decided to take a nursing position on a surgical unit in a community hospital near her home. Mary subsequently told her former colleagues that while she missed the camaraderie she shared with them and the challenges associated with caring for high-risk mothers, she did not miss the stress and profound sadness that was so pervasive in her previous job.

Discussion

This case characterizes the common factors influencing nurse grief. Early in her career, Mary showed numerous signs of empathic engagement. This was validated by the over-recognition shared with her by families. Mary's identification with patients of similar age was most likely related to countertransference; Mary was identifying with patients who were similar to her. A risk associated with this phenomenon is the potential grief that ensues when patients with whom the nurse has a special relationship suffer or die.

Mary was able to persevere in her exemplary holistic nursing care until the magnitude and personal nature of loss hit home. Multiple miscarriages and the death of her mother compounded the degree of Mary's grief. Without giving words to or consciously knowing her reasons why, she withdrew from the more intimate exchanges she historically had with those whom she nursed through critical times. Most likely, a sense of emotional depletion prevailed as a result of her cumulative grief, rendering her unable to nurse in the compassionate manner she had in the past. Mary's professional passion had waned because of her cumulative and unresolved grief. She chose to leave the nursing specialty that initially had offered her much personal and professional reward.

Despair and loss are common in nursing work. The inherent lack of practice-based support diminishes the nurse's capacity for the continued outlay of emotional energy to deal with sorrow. No avenues of support or education were open to Mary to counter the negative effects of her highly affective work. Groups, classes, and individual counseling could have increased Mary's awareness of factors contributing to her growing grief. These supportive measures could have addressed her capacity for introspection and the cultivation of personal hardiness and resilience. At best, the nurse manager making inquiries or Mary sharing her feelings during an exit interview could have generated ideas for work setting improvements. This case represented an example of lost potential resulting from the lack of recognition of supportive interventions with the capacity to influence the longevity and retention of a talented nurse, particularly as it related to her dual mastery of both exemplary biophysiologic and psychosocial patient care.

Notes

References

Bauer, J.J., & Bonanno, G.A. (2001). Continuity amid discontinuity: Bridging one's past and present in stories of conjugal bereavement. *Narrative Inquiry, 11*, 123–158. doi:10.1075/ni.11.1.06bau

Beddoe, A.E., & Murphy, S.O. (2004). Does mindfulness decrease stress and foster empathy among nursing students? *Journal of Nursing Education, 43*, 305–312.

Bonanno, G.A. (2009). *The other side of sadness: What the new science of bereavement tells us about life after loss.* New York, NY: Basic Books.

Bonanno, G.A., & Kaltman, S. (2001). The varieties of grief experience. *Clinical Psychology Review, 21*, 705–734. doi:10.1016/S0272-7358(00)00062-3

Boyle, D.A. (2006). Desperate nursewives [Editorial]. *Oncology Nursing Forum, 33*, 11. doi:10.1188/06.ONF.11

Boyle, D. (2011). Countering compassion fatigue: A requisite nursing agenda. *Online Journal of Issues in Nursing, 16*(1), Manuscript 2. doi:10.3912/OJIN. Vol16No01Man02

Code gray: Care for the caregivers. (2008). *Roswellness, 11*(2), 23. Retrieved from http://www.roswellpark.org/media/publications/roswellness-vol-11-no-2 -summer-08

Di Rado, A. (2009). Tea for the Soul banishes stress and gives caregivers some "me time." *Hope News, 4*(7). Retrieved from http://www.cityofhope.org/ about/publications/hope-news/2009-vol-4-num-7-march-2/Pages/ tea-for-the-soul-banishes-stress-and-gives-caregivers-some-me-time.aspx

Field, N.P., & Horowitz, M.J. (1998). Applying an empty-chair monologue paradigm to examine unresolved grief. *Psychiatry, 61,* 279–287.

Harrison, R.L., & Westwood, M.J. (2009). Preventing vicarious traumatization of mental health therapists: Identifying protective practices. *Psychotherapy, 46,* 203–219. doi:10.1037/a0016081

Holland, J.M., Neimeyer, R.A., Boelen, P.A., & Prigerson, H.G. (2009). The underlying structure of grief: A taxometric investigation of prolonged and normal reactions to loss. *Journal of Psychopathology and Behavior Assessment, 31,* 190–201.

Kearney, M.K., Weininger, R.B., Vachon, M.L.S., Harrison, R.L., & Mount, B.M. (2011). Self-care of physicians caring for patients at the end of life: "Being connected … A key to my survival." In S.J. McPhee, M.A. Winker, M.W. Rabow, S.Z. Pantilat, & A.J. Markowitz (Eds.), *Care at the close of life: Evidence and experience* (pp. 551–562). New York, NY: McGraw-Hill.

Keidel, G.C. (2002). Burnout and compassion fatigue among hospice caregivers. *American Journal of Hospice and Palliative Care, 19,* 200–205. doi:10.1177/104990910201900312

Konigsberg, R.D. (2011). *The truth about grief: The myth of its five stages and the new science of loss.* New York, NY: Simon & Schuster.

Lobb, E.A., Oldham, L., Vojkovic, S., Kristjanson, L.J., Smith, J., Brown, J.M., & Dwyer, V.W. (2010). Frontline grief: The workplace support needs of community palliative care nurses after the death of a patient. *Journal of Hospice and Palliative Nursing, 12,* 234–235. doi:10.1097/NJH.0b013e3181eb07a8

Okun, B., & Nowinski, J. (2011). *Saying goodbye: How families can find renewal through loss.* New York, NY: Berkley Books.

Sherman, D.W. (2004). Nurses' stress and burnout: How to care for yourself when caring for patients and their families experiencing life-threatening illness. *American Journal of Nursing, 104*(5), 48–56.

Sumner, J., & Townsend-Rocchiccioli, J. (2003). Why are nurses leaving nursing? *Nursing Administration Quarterly, 27,* 164–171.

Whitmer, M., Hurst, S., Stadler, K., & Ide, R. (2007). Caring in the curing environment: The implementation of a grieving cart in the ICU. *Journal of Hospice and Palliative Nursing, 9,* 329–333. doi:10.1097/01. NJH.0000299318.30009.f7

Recommended Reading

Albert, P.L. (2001). Grief and loss in the workplace. *Progress in Transplantation, 11,* 169–173.

Notes

Boyle, D.M. (1997). "Coding" the cancer patient: Nurses facilitate family acceptance and grief [Letter]. *Oncology Nursing Forum, 24,* 458.

Brown, C., & Wood, A. (2009). Oncology nurses' grief: A literature review. *Clinical Journal of Oncology Nursing, 13,* 625–627. doi:10.1188/09. CJON.625-627

Brunelli, T. (2005). A concept analysis: The grieving process for nurses. *Nursing Forum, 40,* 123–128. doi:10.1111/j.1744-6198.2005.00024.x

Gerow, L., Conejo, P., Alonzo, A., Davis, N., Rodgers, S., & Domian, E. (2009). A phenomenological study of nurses' experience of grief following patient death. *Western Journal of Nursing Research, 31,* 1078–1079. doi:10.1177/0193945909342243

Greenstreet, W. (2005). Loss, grief and bereavement in interprofessional education, an example of process: Anecdotes and accounts. *Nurse Education in Practice, 5,* 281–288. doi:10.1016/j.nepr.2005.02.003

Keene, E.A., Hutton, N., Hall, B., & Rushton, C. (2010). Bereavement debriefing sessions: An intervention to support health care professionals in managing their grief after the death of a patient. *Pediatric Nursing, 36,* 185–189.

Marino, P.A. (1998). The effects of cumulative grief in the nurse. *Journal of Intravenous Nursing, 21,* 101–104.

McGrath, J.M. (2011). Neonatal nurses: What about their grief and loss? *Journal of Perinatal and Neonatal Nursing, 25,* 8–9. doi:10.1097/JPN.0b013e318208cbf6

Redinbaugh, E.M., Schuerger, J.M., Weiss, L.L., Brufsky, A., & Arnold, R. (2001). Health care professionals' grief: A model based on occupational style and coping. *Psycho-Oncology, 10,* 187–198. doi:10.1002/pon.507

Internet Resources

Growth House: www.growthhouse.org

Medical College of Wisconsin End-of-Life/Palliative Education Resource Center: www.eperc.mcw.edu

University of Massachusetts Medical School Center for Mindfulness in Medicine, Health Care, and Society: www.umassmed.edu/cfm/mbsr

Writing and Health: http://homepage.psy.utexas.edu/homepage/faculty/pennebaker/home2000/writingandhealth.html

Notes

Chapter 6

SPIRITUALITY

Introduction

Nurses often recognize the basic self-care activities that are necessary to prevent or resolve the empathic fatigue syndromes—compassion fatigue, vicarious traumatization, and secondary traumatic stress disorder. These activities include but are not limited to adequate sleep and rest, exercise, good nutrition, and maintaining positive relationships. Yet, many nurses find themselves engulfed in the stressors of their work and personal lives and do not place priority on self-care activities. Why is this? It is proposed that nurses become immobilized or "stuck" and, as experienced in secondary traumatic stress disorder, may actually lose the sense of meaning and purpose in their life. Symptoms of traumatized states are closely aligned with spiritual distress; nurses may feel ungrounded in the world and lose their sense of self.

Spirituality includes everything that helps a person feel connected to something greater than oneself, to a sense of wonder and transcendence in life. It includes faith, spiritual beliefs, religious practices, and a connection to others. Spirituality can bring a sense of order to chaos at a time of existential crisis or search for meaning (Brown-Saltzman, 2009). Spirituality brings *hope*. Spiritual well-being is important for health and for coping with stressful life events; therefore, it is addressed here.

Spirituality is the expression of the mind, body, and spirit (Brown-Saltzman, 1997). Spirituality may be best understood as

Notes

the dimension of being human that motivates self-transcendence and transpersonal interconnectedness (Taylor, 2011). Spirituality can be viewed as the center of one's being. It is the dimension of humanness that prompts people to long for a deeper connection and purpose in life (Taugher, 2002).

It has been written that a spiritual dimension exists in all people and that this dimension integrates and relates to all other dimensions of being human (Taylor, 2006). "At the core of the spiritual dimension is the drive to find the meaning in life's experiences" (Musgrave & McFarlane, 2003, p. 523). Spirituality connects us to our place within the world, to our relationships within it, to the community, and to nature.

Why is spirituality important? Spirituality is a major component of holistic nursing care (Delaney, 2005) and is important for nurses and patients alike. Tapping into one's spirituality promotes self-healing and may be a preventive measure against burnout and compassion fatigue. Spiritual well-being also helps nurses connect to the powerful meaning of their work (Brown-Saltzman, 2009). Deep spiritual reflection is a coping resource that may allow nurses to be present in the suffering of others (Ferrell & Coyle, 2008). The literature has also shown that nurses who connect with their own spirituality are more likely to provide spiritual care to their patients (Taylor, 2006).

Spirituality is an awakening to what is significant in life; it allows individuals to lean on something greater than themselves (Brown-Saltzman, 2009). Contrary to spirituality, *religion* has been defined as an "organized set of practices that surround a traditionally defined belief in the existence of God or divine sacred writings and a set of rituals used to express or practice beliefs" (Taugher, 2002, p. 239). Spirituality is a component of religious beliefs or practices, but religious practices or beliefs may or may not be a part of spirituality (Taugher, 2002). Research has shown a link between spiritual well-being and religiosity (Musgrave & McFarlane, 2004), but practice of an organized religion is not necessary for spiritual beliefs. Spirituality is expanded from a relationship with God or a "higher being" to self, community, and an environment that nurtures and celebrates wholeness (Musgrave & McFarlane, 2003).

Taylor (2011) outlined a health psychology framework that supports the role of spirituality and health (see Figure 8). If nurses honor the sacred in life, they may honor the sacredness of their own bodies, leading to choosing healthy lifestyle behaviors and self-care activities. Thus, spirituality is important for both physical and mental health.

Figure 8. Spirituality and Health

- Spirituality creates a sense of meaning and purpose.
- Social support, which is part of a faith community, is linked to health.
- Sacredness of body and health leads to positive lifestyle behaviors.
- How people believe that they or God controls their health may have an impact on health behaviors.
- Components of spirituality—gratitude, hope, optimism, and compassion—contribute to a sense of meaningfulness and social connection.
- Behaviors such as prayer and meditation have stress-buffering effects.
- Positive religious coping has a stress-buffering effect.

Note. Based on information from Taylor, 2011.

Notes

REFLECTION

Do you consider yourself spiritual or religious? _____

_____

Do you have spiritual beliefs that help you cope with stress? _____

_____

_____

What gives your life meaning and purpose? _____

_____

_____

(Continued on next page)

REFLECTION *(CONTINUED)*

What importance does your faith or beliefs play in your life? _____
_____
_____

Have your beliefs influenced how you take care of yourself?_____
_____
_____

Are you a part of a religious or spiritual community? Is this supportive to you, and if so, how? _____
_____
_____

Is there a group of people you love or who are really important to you? _____
_____
_____

Who are your greatest support systems?_____
_____
_____

Do you carry out practices to support your spirituality (e.g., meditation, prayer, yoga)? _____
_____
_____

Do you utilize your spirituality when you give care to your patients? _____
_____
_____

Note. Based on information from Puchalski, 2006; Puchalski & Romer, 2000.

Spirituality is looking inward for answers and involves reflection, enabling nurses to care for themselves and others. It is listening to one's inner voice to find meaning (Loney & Murphy-Ende, 2009). Brown-Saltzman (1994) asked whether it is even possible to do the work of nursing without some spiritual connection. It is important for nurses to identify the spiritual element within themselves before they can provide spiritual care to others in need. Research has found an association between nurses' spiritual well-being and positive attitudes toward spiritual care: "Nurses who have high levels of spiritual well-being may be more aware of their own spirituality and, therefore, more open to discern their patients' spiritual concerns" (Musgrave & McFarlane, 2003, p. 527). Nurses also must acknowledge the diversity of spiritual and religious beliefs and that the meaning of spirituality is individualized. Taugher (2002) encouraged nurses to understand that patients become frustrated at their inability to overcome the limitations of their lives or their illness, and that they want to know that these feelings do not go unnoticed by those near and dear to them. Patients may find that spirituality is a comfort during their illness or that a life-threatening diagnosis spins them into a spiritual crisis, causing them to search for the meaning of their illness within the context of their lives. In summary, nurses who have defined their own spirituality are more likely to help patients through their life crises. To stay present in the emotional anguish and suffering of others, nurses often need to rely on inner reflection and their own spirituality (Ferrell & Coyle, 2008).

No other area of nursing may test a nurse's spirituality more than palliative care, where caregivers are challenged to work through their own emotions and grief related to the care of dying patients. In one study on palliative care, self-healing in the midst of suffering emerged as an unspoken potential when working with dying patients (Mulder & Gregory, 2000). Compassion and loving kindness were seen as transforming the nurse into a genuine healer. One nurse expressed that her journey provided her with a sense of who she was and a deeper understanding of what life and death meant to her (Mulder & Gregory, 2000). Spirituality has been described as the "fuel" that restores nurses' unique ability to continue meeting the needs of dying patients and their families (Loney & Murphy-Ende, 2009). Yet, the spiritual distress of witnessing suffering may cause a crisis of faith in the nurse's own life (Brown-Saltzman, 2009).

Notes

REFLECTION

Spirituality Scale

The Spirituality Scale may be self-administered to assess one's own level of spirituality. Please indicate your level of agreement to the following statements by circling the appropriate number that corresponds with the answer key:

1 = Strongly disagree
2 = Disagree
3 = Mostly disagree
4 = Mostly agree
5 = Agree
6 = Strongly agree

1. I find meaning in my life experiences.	1 2 3 4 5 6
2. I have a sense of purpose.	1 2 3 4 5 6
3. I am happy about the person I have become.	1 2 3 4 5 6
4. I see the sacredness in everyday life.	1 2 3 4 5 6
5. I meditate to gain access to my inner spirit.	1 2 3 4 5 6
6. I live in harmony with nature.	1 2 3 4 5 6
7. I believe there is a connection between all things that I cannot see but can sense.	1 2 3 4 5 6
8. My life is a process of becoming.	1 2 3 4 5 6
9. I believe in a Higher Power/Universal Intelligence.	1 2 3 4 5 6
10. I believe that all living creatures deserve respect.	1 2 3 4 5 6
11. The earth is sacred.	1 2 3 4 5 6
12. I value maintaining and nurturing my relationships with others.	1 2 3 4 5 6
13. I use silence to get in touch with myself.	1 2 3 4 5 6

(Continued on next page)

REFLECTION *(CONTINUED)*	
14. I believe that nature should be respected.	1 2 3 4 5 6
15. I have a relationship with a Higher Power/Universal Intelligence.	1 2 3 4 5 6
16. My spirituality gives me inner strength.	1 2 3 4 5 6
17. I am able to receive love from others.	1 2 3 4 5 6
18. My faith in a Higher Power/Universal Intelligence helps me cope during challenges in my life.	1 2 3 4 5 6
19. I strive to correct the excesses in my own lifestyle patterns/practices.	1 2 3 4 5 6
20. I respect the diversity of people.	1 2 3 4 5 6
21. Prayer is an integral part of my spiritual nature.	1 2 3 4 5 6
22. At times, I feel at one with the universe.	1 2 3 4 5 6
23. I often take time to assess my life choices as a way of living my spirituality.	1 2 3 4 5 6

Scoring of Spirituality Scale

23–60	Low level of spirituality; spiritual distress
61–91	Low level of spirituality; possible spiritual distress
92–117	Moderate spirituality; potential for spiritual distress
118–138	High level of spirituality; spiritual wellness

Note. Based on information from Delaney, 2005.

Notes

Interventions

Interventions that replenish the spirit are crucial for nurses suffering from burnout or one of the empathic syndromes. Research has demonstrated that spiritual well-being is an indicator of spiritual health; therefore, nurses who can identify their own spiritual distress may be alerted to seek spiritual counseling. Brown-Saltzman (1997) asserted that spiritual caregiving prevents burnout. Stebnicki (2008) stated that spiritual care drives to the core of our very being and is an essential part of healing empathy fatigue. "Using spiritual practices enhances well-being, connects individuals to the community, and helps them to cope" (Brown-Saltzman, 2009, p. 232).

Spirituality is a source of inspiration, creativity, and wisdom (Loney & Murphy-Ende, 2009). Replenishing the spirit comes from finding meaning for oneself and "feeling the connectivity and transcendence that takes us beyond our limited and imaginary control" (Brown-Saltzman, 1997, p. 258). Guided imagery is an example of a spiritual practice that uses imagination to instill a state of relaxation and calmness. Any of the spiritual practices outlined in Figure 9 can give the nurse a sense of control and tranquility. Creativity in the form of art, music, dance, journaling, or other outlets can provide what Brown-Saltzman (2009) referred to as the *healing path.*

In a very busy schedule of work and other responsibilities, spiritual self-care may seem daunting. Yet, touching one's spiritual self can begin with the simple exercise of stopping for one minute per day to take a deep breath, feeling the energy of life as you inhale. It may begin by taking a few minutes a day to feel the sun on your face or to notice a rainbow after a storm. The spirit is closely tied to nature—simply walking in a garden can bring about a sense of awe and gratitude. When nurses find connection to creation and a sense of wonder, this spirituality helps to bring meaning and balance in their personal and professional lives (Brown-Saltzman, 2009). Brown-Saltzman (1994) eloquently stated that when the spirit is tended to within the person, then the cry of pain cannot be ignored and the person can no longer squelch his or her own needs.

Figure 9. Self-Care to Enhance Spirituality

- Activities and cognitive reframing that create meaningfulness
  - Altruistic activities (i.e., unselfish acts of kindness)
  - Dedication to a scientific, social, religious, or political cause
  - Hedonistic activities (i.e., highly pleasurable activities)
- Experiences that allow self-expression or enhance self-understanding
  - Visual arts
  - Literature (e.g., writing poetry, bibliotherapy)
  - Journal writing
  - Music
  - Kinesthetic arts (e.g., dance)
  - Other "art" forms (e.g., cooking, flower arranging)
- Dream analysis (i.e., exploring the significance of dreams, learning about the spiritual life by being attentive to messages found in dreams)
- Forgiveness therapy
- Religious or nonreligious rituals
- Meditation and prayer
- Being with nature
- Reading sacred writings or other spiritual material
- Storytelling (i.e., life review)
- Presencing (i.e., being there, being fully present)
- Consulting with spiritual care experts (e.g., clergy, spiritual counselor, chaplain)

Note. From "Spirituality and Spiritual Nurture in Cancer Care" (p. 124), by E.J. Taylor in R.M. Carroll-Johnson, L.M. Gorman, and N.J. Bush (Eds.), *Psychosocial Nursing Care Along the Cancer Continuum* (2nd ed.), 2006, Pittsburgh, PA: Oncology Nursing Society. Copyright 2006 by the Oncology Nursing Society. Reprinted with permission.

Notes

Delaney (2005) recommended interventions to support findings on the Spirituality Scale (shown in the previous Reflection). Self-care activities such as reflection, journaling, listening to music, meditation, and relaxation techniques enhance the existential component of spirituality and serve as a bridge to self-discovery. Relationships are another inherent component of spirituality. Building healthy relationships can be achieved through counseling, participation in support groups, engagement with family, friends, and colleagues, and even experiencing energy therapies (e.g., Reiki) to bring into consciousness the interconnectedness of life. Lastly, nurses can nurture the relationship of spirituality

Notes

to nature by the creation of caring environments, spending more time in natural settings that are perceived to be healing, and surrounding oneself with nature through plants and art therapy.

Aycock and Boyle (2009) discussed the following ways in which nurses can expand self-care into the spiritual realm.

- **Saying good-bye to patients.** Closure with patients and families is an often-overlooked entity in the clinical setting. Nurses grieve the loss of their patients; they are also in the circle of the bereaved. Interventions must be individualized to provide comfort in accordance with the nurse's belief system but may include attending a patient's funeral, writing sympathy cards, or displaying memories on bulletin boards. These activities can support individual and staff grief and loss.

- **Pastoral care.** The clinical chaplain and pastoral care staff can provide ceremonial opportunities to support nurses. These activities may include support groups after a death or ceremonies such as a "blessing of hands" for staff members. Routine availability of pastoral care for patients and families also will reassure nursing staff that the special needs of their patients are being met.

- **Retreats.** Annual or biannual retreats can prove to be beneficial by providing nurses with respite from the intensity of work. Conducted off-site, retreats can provide nurses with a safe haven to partner with nature, meditate, journal, share feelings with supportive peers, or stimulate healing through art, music, and guided imagery.

- **Counseling.** The ideal would be to have a counselor or psychologist who is assigned to each unit of care and is available for both patients and staff. If this is not possible, ongoing support services can take place on a regular basis outside of the normative "staff meeting." Nurses who work with high-acuity patients or those with life-threatening illnesses warrant a safe and peaceful forum in which to share feelings and divulge grief.

As a strategy to retain oncology nurses and as a forum for healing, nurses at Brigham and Women's Hospital in Boston, Massachusetts, created a program called Spirit Rounds (Hayes et al., 2005). The inpatient facility initiated Spirit Rounds to provide the nurses with a vehicle to examine difficult issues encountered in their compassionate care of patients with cancer. "Supporting patients and families as they struggle to live with cancer diagnoses, hope for remission, or cope with dying and death can leave oncology nurses emotionally depleted" (Hayes et al., 2005, p. 1089). The goals of Spirit Rounds were to provide a safe haven for the nurses to talk about the caring relationships they developed with their patients, to share feelings about patient encounters, to offer emotional support to each other, and to reconnect with the compassion and spirituality inherent in oncology nursing. An important outcome was to create an opportunity for staff to also explore the relationships they had with each other (Hayes et al., 2005). The idea of Spirit Rounds could be applied in both inpatient and outpatient settings and can serve as a means to bring the interdisciplinary team together on a consistent basis to provide mutual support and a safe arena in which to share feelings of spiritual distress. Other major issues that fall under the realm of spiritual concerns could also be addressed, for example, ethics. "Another aspect of human spirituality is the moral side of life. A person's inner being is not only psychological and emotional but moral as well" (Taugher, 2002, p. 239) (see Chapter 7).

Summary

Spiritual well-being has demonstrated a positive relationship with both physical and mental health. Spirituality is important to prevent and resolve the empathic syndromes, and symptoms of spiritual distress are closely aligned with the symptoms of compassion fatigue, vicarious traumatization, and secondary traumatic stress disorder. Nurses who are able to identify their own belief systems may be more likely to carry out self-care behaviors, and these nurses are more likely to incorporate spiritual care into their work.

Case Study

Cindy had worked as an advanced practice nurse (APN) on the oncology unit of her community hospital for many years. Al-

Notes

though this specialized area often was emotionally stressful, Cindy always felt positive regarding the contributions she made to the quality of life of her patients. She also relished her relationships with her colleagues and used her position as an APN to promote a supportive environment for the staff. Although Cindy worked many hours of overtime a day, often without adequate breaks for rest or meals, she seemed to run on the pure energy that her work supplied her. Cindy always felt rewarded by her accomplishments with patients and staff. Although she did not take time for reflection or self-care activities outside of work, she always felt she had strong coping techniques to deal with any stress or adversity that challenged her.

Recently, a routine mammogram showed that Cindy had a nodule in her left breast. Because the tumor was found in its early stages, Cindy felt genuinely positive about her prognosis. Although node negative, Cindy's tumor was multifocal, and ductal carcinoma in situ was found in the surrounding breast tissue. This and her premenopausal status indicated the need for a mastectomy with reconstruction and six cycles of prophylactic chemotherapy. As the process of her treatment unfolded, Cindy remained optimistic about her ability to cope with both her diagnosis and the treatment. She thought that because she had always inspired courage and positive spirit in her patients, she herself could be as brave.

Cindy was divorced and responsible for raising her three young children. Because of the demands of her APN work and her young children at home, Cindy decided to take a leave of absence from her job to focus on her health and well-being. She also needed to balance the demands of her treatment with her responsibilities as a single mother. Her adolescent daughter could help take care of the two younger sons, but because her former husband had minimum childcare involvement, taking care of her children now necessitated more of her energy during treatment.

Cindy proved to be strong both physically and mentally throughout her six months of treatment, all the while positive that she would return to her APN job when treatment was completed. In fact, in some ways she cherished the time with her family and was grateful for the time off from the stressors at work. She knew she could not have kept up the pace of her job while bat-tling the disease and undergoing treatment.

Upon completion of therapy, Cindy was stunned to find her-self physically and emotionally drained. When she got the "clean bill of health" to return to her job, she found that she couldn't do it. She asked herself how she could keep up with the emotion-al needs of the patients, their families, and the staff while at the same time trying to take care of her own. Cindy doubted that she would be able to return to work and keep up with the fast pace and demands of her position—she was having a hard time keep-ing up with the needs of her children. Cindy felt overwhelming fatigue after treatment. When she decided to resign from the job she had loved so much, she began to feel a sense of loss.

Cindy made no effort to find another job immediately. She felt that her health and recovery were the most important priori-ties next to the care of her children. She also felt that she would steadily regain her strength and move forward with another job opportunity, given her skills and years of experience. Yet, as the months passed, Cindy found that her fatigue lingered along with residual effects of her treatment and the chemotherapy-induced menopause. Cindy suffered from peripheral neuropathies, hot flashes, insomnia, mood changes, and an overwhelming anxiety that she couldn't pinpoint. She began to have flashbacks not only of her treatment but also of the patients she had cared for during her oncology work. Many times she would wake up startled with shortness of breath, having dreamed of a beloved patient she had lost. Or she would dream about losing her own battle against can-cer, as she had witnessed so many times in her work setting. Fol-low-up examinations became triggers. As she became tired of peo-ple she encountered inquiring about her illness, Cindy began to withdraw into herself. Although she had close family and friends, she found that they seemed to have moved back into their lives and expected her to do the same. Cindy felt like a different per-son than before and even began to question her ability to return to her oncology work. She resented that she had become ill and found herself asking questions like, "Why me?" and "Why *not* me?" She also began to doubt her faith. Why would God have asked her to take this journey, when her life was devoted to helping and car-

Notes

ing for others? Now she felt alone and in despair. Overall, Cindy began to feel a sense of numbness and estrangement from even her family and close friends. She constantly asked herself, "What is the meaning of my life?"

Discussion

After her cancer treatment ended, Cindy was showing symptoms of secondary traumatic stress disorder. Her own traumatic experience was bringing forth unresolved traumas from her previous work. She was having flashbacks and nightmares of not only herself but her patients as well. Cindy did not start her cancer journey on strong footing. Her previous job had drained many of her physical and emotional resources. She felt much personal reward from her work, but she ignored any self-care or healing strategies needed to maintain her health prior to her diagnosis. Although she was courageous and relied on the life lessons she had learned from her patients, Cindy had unresolved trauma from both her personal and professional life.

Cindy also began to isolate herself to avoid reminders of her recent journey, as people who asked her about her health were triggers bringing forth the grief and loss she had experienced from her disease and treatment. Follow-up examinations also served as a reminder of what she was now feeling as a painful journey. Cindy was also questioning whether she could return to her oncology work because patients' diagnoses of cancer may trigger her anxiety and fear.

Cindy is experiencing an existential or spiritual crisis. She doubts her faith, and after resigning from her position as an APN and struggling with the residual effects of cancer treatment, she feels lost in her sense of purpose. Cindy was questioning the meaning of life when asking "Why me?" and "Why not me?" The time for therapeutic intervention for Cindy is now. This could be in the form of individual or group psychotherapy. Cindy needs help to tap into the unresolved traumas that are affecting her worldview. As she confronts the symptoms of traumatic stress disorder, Cindy may be able to find meaning in her cancer journey and also resolve the impact that her work has and will have on her new identity. As Cindy moves forward, she will need to integrate a new meaning and purpose into her changed life. This will include deciding whether to return to the same type of work at this time. Therapeutic intervention also should incorporate self-reflective activities for Cindy, such as meditation, journaling, and other creative outlets. If Cindy is involved in a faith community, it would be advantageous for her to speak with a spiritual counselor or minister.

Cindy is currently in danger of becoming immobilized by her anxiety or developing depression if she continues to isolate herself without any means of communicating her deep feelings and fears (see Chapters 8 and 9). Therapeutic intervention is necessary for Cindy to heal spiritually.

References

Aycock, N., & Boyle, D. (2009). Interventions to manage compassion fatigue in oncology nursing. *Clinical Journal of Oncology Nursing, 13,* 183–191. doi:10.1188/09.CJON.183-191

Brown-Saltzman, K.A. (1994). Tending the spirit. *Oncology Nursing Forum, 21,* 1001–1006.

Brown-Saltzman, K. (1997). Replenishing the spirit by meditative prayer and guided imagery. *Seminars in Oncology Nursing, 13,* 255–259. doi:10.1016/S0749-2081(97)80021-6

Brown-Saltzman, K. (2009). Self-care for nurses. In C.C. Burke (Ed.), *Psychosocial dimensions of oncology nursing care* (2nd ed., pp. 217–244). Pittsburgh, PA: Oncology Nursing Society.

Delaney, C. (2005). The Spirituality Scale: Development and psychometric testing of a holistic instrument to assess the human spiritual dimension. *Journal of Holistic Nursing, 23,* 145–167. doi:10.1177/0898010105276180

Ferrell, B.R., & Coyle, N. (2008). The nature of suffering and the goals of nursing. *Oncology Nursing Forum, 35,* 241–247. doi:10.1188/08.ONF.241-247

Hayes, C., Ponte, P.R., Coakley, A., Stanghellini, E., Gross, A., Perryman, S., … Somerville, J. (2005). Retaining oncology nurses: Strategies for today's nurse leaders. *Oncology Nursing Forum, 32,* 1087–1090. doi:10.1188/05.ONF.1087-1090

Loney, M., & Murphy-Ende, K. (2009). Death, dying, and grief in the face of cancer. In C.C. Burke (Ed.), *Psychosocial dimensions of oncology nursing care* (2nd ed., pp. 159–185). Pittsburgh, PA: Oncology Nursing Society.

Mulder, J., & Gregory, D. (2000). Transforming experience into wisdom: Healing amidst suffering. *Journal of Palliative Care, 16*(2), 25–29.

Musgrave, C.F., & McFarlane, E.A. (2003). Oncology and nononcology nurses' spiritual well-being and attitudes toward spiritual care: A literature review. *Oncology Nursing Forum, 30,* 523–527. doi:10.1188/03.ONF.523-527

Notes

Musgrave, C.F., & McFarlane, E.A. (2004). Israeli oncology nurses' religiosity, spiritual well-being, and attitudes toward spiritual care: A path analysis. *Oncology Nursing Forum, 31,* 321–327. doi:10.1188/04.ONF.321-327

Puchalski, C. (2006). Spiritual assessment in clinical practice. *Psychiatric Annals, 36,* 150–155.

Puchalski, C., & Romer, A.L. (2000). Taking a spiritual history allows clinicians to understand patients more fully. *Journal of Palliative Medicine, 3,* 129–137. doi:10.1089/jpm.2000.3.129

Stebnicki, M.A. (2008). *Empathy fatigue: Healing the mind, body, and spirit of professional counselors.* New York, NY: Springer.

Taugher, T. (2002). Helping patients search for meaning in their lives. *Clinical Journal of Oncology Nursing, 6,* 239–240. doi:10.1188/02.CJON.239-240

Taylor, E.J. (2006). Spirituality and spiritual nurture in cancer care. In R.M. Carroll-Johnson, L.M. Gorman, & N.J. Bush (Eds.), *Psychosocial nursing care along the cancer continuum* (2nd ed., pp. 117–131). Pittsburgh, PA: Oncology Nursing Society.

Taylor, E.J. (2011). Spiritual responses to cancer. In C.H. Yarbro, D. Wujcik, & B.H. Gobel (Eds.), *Cancer nursing: Principles and practice* (7th ed., pp. 1797–1812). Sudbury, MA: Jones and Bartlett.

Recommended Reading

Levine, S. (2005). *Unattended sorrow: Recovering from loss and reviving the heart.* Emmaus, PA: Rodale.

Sulmasy, D.P. (1997). *The healer's calling: A spirituality for physicians and other health care professionals.* New York, NY: Paulist Press.

Internet Resources

FICA Assessment: Taking a Spiritual History: www.mentalhealthministries.net/links_resources/other_resources/fica_assessment.pdf

Spirituality and Practice, Resources for Spiritual Journeys: www.spiritualityandpractice.com

Notes

MORAL DISTRESS

Introduction

Today's healthcare environment is exemplified by rapid change, an evolving acute care patient population, and workplace limitations in both staff and resources. An explosion of technologic advances, heightened patient acuity in tandem with the greater chronicity of many illnesses, cost containment measures, regulatory oversight, staffing constraints, ineffective leadership, and a rise in the percentage of older adult patients presents numerous dilemmas for nurses and their colleagues. Of major concern is how these trends influence the rendering of ethically sound patient care.

Although the terms *ethics* and *morals* often are used interchangeably, they characterize two distinct yet interrelated entities. *Ethics* is a formal, theoretical term that refers to a publicly stated set of rules or values embraced by a designated group. *Morals*, on the other hand, is a more informal term that refers to a set of personal values or principles to which an individual ascribes. Both of these phenomena become important when differences arise that influence how nursing care is delivered, both in the context of medical decision making and the highly individualized delivery of patient care.

Witnessing patient struggle and suffering (of both an intrapsychic and physical nature) often is associated with conflict for nurses. Usually, some corollary of dying and death is the genesis of this contention. For critical care nurses, moral distress situations frequently involve disparity in judgment regarding continuation of aggressive therapy (McClendon & Buckner, 2007). Pendry (2007) termed this phenomenon *dueling expectations.*

Several professional caregiver qualities influence discord surrounding issues of conscience. Astuteness and sensitivity to religiosity and cultural orientation are paramount in any deliberation involving ethical or moral questioning. These phenomena significantly influence patient and family decision making, particularly at the end of life. Patients bring to the medical encounter different languages, explanatory models concerning the causes and treatment of illness, and an interpretation of dying and death that may differ from the professional caregiver's. What frequently results is elevation of the caregiver's beliefs and values and negation of the patient's. For example, nurses may "problematize" spiritual aspects of a patient's care, categorizing them as ethical problems (e.g., code status, futility) or as psychosocial sequelae (e.g., denial) (Kagawa-Singer & Blackhall, 2011). Other corollaries of health professionals' responses to ethical dilemmas include their knowledge of ethical principles and previous experience with unethical behavior.

Numerous ethical constructs have relevance for nurses. *Moral uncertainty* is exemplified by unease and questioning when the nurse is unclear about the appropriate course of action. A *moral dilemma* is evident when the nurse perceives conflicting but morally justifiable avenues of action and questions which is best for the patient. *Moral distress* characterizes a state of painful psychological disequilibrium (some even refer to it as suffering) that results from recognizing the ethically appropriate action, yet not acting on it. In short, it is the inability to translate moral choices into moral action (Rushton, 2006). Internal or external constraints (e.g., lack of time, supervisory reluctance, an inhibiting medical power structure, institutional policy, legal considerations) may impede or prevent healthcare providers from taking the action they believe is right. Moral distress can contribute to substandard workplace practices. Nurses may avoid particular patients or engage in poor communication with coworkers, which can erode teamwork and interdisciplinary cohesion (Robinson, 2010). Evidence of moral distress usually is a sign that ethical challenges are not being adequately addressed, and the provision of optimum patient care is at risk (Epstein & Delgado, 2010). Moral distress likes to prey on nurses (Unruh, 2010). Nurse vulnerability can be directly correlated with two prominent attributes: the intimate nature of nursing work and the nurse's role as patient advocate. Nurses' relationships with patients are grounded on understanding and confidentiality. This then fosters a unique sense of knowing the patient. Nurses also uniformly embrace the responsibility to be the voice of patients, particularly when circumstances prevent patients from speaking for themselves. Prominent antecedents of moral distress include conflicting opinions between nurses and physicians and between nurses and families, particularly with situations involving end-of-life decision making or the provision of futile care. Certain managed care directives and rationed care constraints are examples of fiscal corollaries of moral distress. Of note is the contemporary variable of *moral residue,* a consequence of unresolved moral distress. It is the end result of compromise, a violation of moral values caused by constraints beyond the nurse's control.

Rendering nursing care within this context of moral challenge can prompt stress responses in staff manifested in the form of psychosomatic complaints such as insomnia, anxiety, headaches, or gastrointestinal distress. The internalization of moral anguish may provoke coping responses such as anger, guilt, remorse, blaming (self or others), self-criticism, and the use of avoidance behaviors. Staff members may report extreme sadness and tearfulness and feel embarrassed and confused by feelings of despondency. When no outlet exists in which to discuss or attempt to resolve the nature of moral distress, intra- and interdisciplinary conflict prevails. Staff may exhibit chronic discontent, passive-aggressive behavior, absenteeism, and decreased productivity within the workplace. Abusive behaviors may surface. Nurses may change or transfer positions or ultimately leave the profession.

Notes

REFLECTION

Answer the following questions.

On a 0–10 scale, rate how pervasive moral distress is in your practice setting.
Score: ___   Describe why you gave that rating and give supporting examples.

_____

_____

What situations cause the greatest degree of moral distress?

_____

_____

How does moral distress affect the delivery of nursing care in your practice setting?

_____

_____

What could be implemented in your work setting to help nurses better cope with moral distress? Specify three things:

_____

_____

_____

On a 0–10 scale, rate your overall level of moral distress.
Score: ___   Describe why you gave that rating.

_____

_____

How does moral distress affect your work performance? How does your nursing change when moral distress prevails?

_____

_____

How does workplace-related moral distress affect your personal life?

_____

_____

These reflections can be shared in a group setting with a facilitator who guides the discussion, pointing out similarities or themes that evolve. The discussion should end with consensus on possible interventions to implement in the practice setting to reduce the prevalence of moral distress. Consider easy, practical interventions to begin. Lobbying for enhanced human resources in the work setting, for example, will take significant negotiation, planning, and time.

Interventions

Concern about worker safety and well-being is a growing trend throughout the United States. Recognition of the healthcare environment as being stressful and potentially unsafe has driven the assimilation of workplace interventions to promote employee wellness. Such programs include the provision of on-site exercise centers, nutritional consultation for staff, and complimentary services for stress reduction, such as yoga and massage therapy. Both managers and staff must assume responsibility for the creation, viability, and sustainability of worksite wellness programs. Healthcare organizations can promote ethical fitness in their employees through education, role-modeling, and access to expert resources and consultants. Ensuring that frontline nurses are appointed to key committees that influence ethical practices will enhance organizational sensitivity and orientation to moral distress issues (Pendry, 2007). The promotion of moral courage is paramount. It is the epitome of ethical behavior whereby individuals maintain their resolve to "do the right thing" despite the potential negative consequences they may face, such as threats to personal reputation, isolation, retaliation, or loss of employment (Murray, 2010).

Notes

REFLECTION

Certain organizational characteristics have the potential to impede morally courageous actions. Consider the six inhibitors below (Murray, 2010) relative to your current work setting. Put an X to the left of the statements that are prominent within your work setting.

___ 1. Organizational culture stifles discussion regarding unethical behaviors and tolerates unethical acts.

___ 2. Colleagues are generally willing to compromise personal and professional standards in order to avoid social isolation from peers or to secure a promotion or favoritism within the organization.

___ 3. The environment promotes indifference to ethical values (i.e., as exemplified by coworkers and management).

___ 4. Apathy is exhibited by colleagues who lack the moral courage to take action.

___ 5. "Group think" supports a united decision to "turn the other way" when unethical behaviors are taking place.

___ 6. The tendency to redefine unethical behaviors is acceptable.

Notes

Of note is that while moral distress most certainly has negative corollaries, it also may have positive outcomes in that it increases nurses' awareness of ethical problems (Corley, 2002). It may prompt the construct of *moral courage*, which reflects the nurse's willingness to address an ethical concern or problem that others are sidestepping or ignoring (Lachman, 2007). This is part of the larger paradigm of *moral agency*, an intrinsic philosophy representing nurses' awareness of the worth of their practice (Pask, 2003).

In 2008, the American Association of Critical-Care Nurses revised its position statement identifying moral distress as a significant yet underrecognized problem in nursing. This statement delineated employer imperatives to ameliorate moral distress engendered by critical care nurses. Key points included the following recommendations for organizations.

- Implement interdisciplinary strategies to recognize and name the experience of moral distress.
- Establish mechanisms to monitor the clinical and organizational climate to identify recurring situations that result in moral distress.
- Develop a systematic process for reviewing and analyzing the system issues enabling situations that cause moral distress to occur and for taking corrective action.
- Create support systems that include
  - Employee assistance programs
  - Protocols for end-of-life care
  - Ethics committees
  - Critical stress debriefings
  - Grief counseling.
- Create interdisciplinary forums to discuss patient goals of care and divergent opinions in an open, respectful environment.
- Develop policies that support unobstructed access to resources such as ethics committees.
- Ensure nurses' representation on institutional ethics committees with full participation in decision making.
- Provide education and tools to manage and decrease moral distress in the work environment.

REFLECTION

Consider how many of the following options are available to you. Place an X to the left of the variables that currently exist in your work setting.

___ Presence of an open communication style or forum to discuss patient care issues
___ Regularly scheduled interdisciplinary rounds to review patient status
___ Possibility for generating patient care conferences to discuss "difficult" patients
___ Existence of an employee assistance program
___ Availability of a clinical nurse specialist, counselor, social worker, or pastoral care chaplain to discuss patient scenarios of concern
___ Presence of an ethics committee to assist with ethical decision making
___ Education on ethics and moral distress in orientation and continuing education offerings
___ Availability of a colleague with additional training or expertise in ethics
___ Interdisciplinary family meetings to discuss patient status and prognosis
___ Presence of a palliative care team
___ Shared governance structure in which new program ideas for the unit can be discussed
___ "Open-door" policy of the nurse manager to express concerns or discuss possible unit improvements

If after reviewing the results of this exercise you feel you are limited in needed resources, use the information in this chapter to lobby for additional support.

Summary

This chapter described the concept of moral distress and its corollaries and consequences. The reflective exercises presented will help nurses to identify personal and organizational inventories of moral distress. Nurses should explore potential interventions appropriate for their work setting.

Case Study

Mr. H, a 79-year-old widower whom Julie cared for just three months earlier on the telemetry unit, was admitted again with progressive shortness of breath and dyspnea and tachycardia related to his worsening congestive heart failure and chronic obstructive pulmonary disease. A diagnostic workup revealed a significant reduction in Mr. H's cardiac ejection fraction and multiple QRS interval abnormalities on his electrocardiogram. Despite vasodilators, diuretics, and continuous oxygen therapy, Mr. H remained symptomatic. While Julie was getting him comfortable in bed, in a much-labored manner he shared with her, "I can't live any more like this. I'm ready to go." Julie waited for a moment in silence to determine if Mr. H wanted to talk more about his feelings. She then queried Mr. H about having an advance directive and whether his family knew his wishes. He stated that he did not have a formal written document but that he had discussed several times with his son about wanting no heroics.

Mr. H's son arrived on the unit and asked to speak with the nurse caring for this father. In talking with him, Julie suggested that he connect with the social worker to get the advance directive completed. The son said he was uncomfortable doing this despite his conversations with his father. However, he reluctantly agreed to speak with the social worker. Soon after, Mr. H's primary physician arrived on the unit. Julie brought up the absence of the advance directive and the need to have this conversation with the patient. The physician said he would address it with him in the morning.

Just prior to the end of visiting hours that day, Mr. H was struggling to get up and go into the bathroom with his son's help when he experienced a cardiac arrest. His son screamed for the nurse and yelled, "Help! My father's not breathing—please don't let him die!" A code was called, and Mr. H was ultimately placed on a ventilator and transferred to the intensive care unit.

The next evening, Julie asked a colleague to watch her patients for 30 minutes so she could make a brief visit to the intensive care unit to see how Mr. H was doing. Mr. H's son was in the room holding his father's hand. He was happy to see Julie and thanked her for coming to visit. Julie asked the son if she could have a moment with him outside. In the context of the conversation, she inquired whether he had siblings or a representative of the clergy who could support him during this difficult time. She also relayed the specifics of the short conversation Mr. H had had with her about how he wanted to die. Julie determined the son's receptiveness to speaking to the hospital chaplain, social worker, and primary physician in a family conference to determine what was best for Mr. H. The son agreed to do this upon the arrival of his sister from out of town. Following a subsequent family conference, it was decided to remove

Mr. H from the ventilator. Mr. H's son and daughter, the hospital chaplain, and the intensive care unit nurse were in the room when Mr. H died. Julie made a mental note to speak with her nurse manager next week about this scenario to discuss whether additional resources could be employed upon hospital admission to assist with the proactive determination of advance directives.

Discussion

Julie demonstrated moral courage and the capacity to enact her core values and ethical obligations to her patient. Although the ideal goal was not met (i.e., the initial elimination of heroic measures per patient request), Julie continued to lobby for Mr. H's rights with both his son and physician. Recognizing the potential isolation Mr. H's son felt and the enormity of his decision-making responsibility, the nurse acknowledged his need for support. Her referral to the social worker and chaplain and her suggestion for a family conference demonstrated the existence of workplace resources to counter moral distress. They also minimized the likelihood that prolonged moral conflict would prevail and reduced the likelihood of moral residue, an enduring sense that the nurse didn't do all she could for Mr. H. Her projected plan to discuss this scenario with her nurse manager was indicative of the American Association of Critical-Care Nurses' key recommendation to address recurring situations that result in moral distress for nurses.

References

American Association of Critical-Care Nurses. (2008). Moral distress [Position statement]. Retrieved from http://www.aacn.org/WD/Practice/Docs/Moral_distress.pdf

Corley, M.C. (2002). Nurse moral distress: A proposed theory and research agenda. *Nursing Ethics, 9,* 636–650. doi:10.1191/0969733002ne557oa

Epstein, E.G., & Delgado, S. (2010). Understanding and addressing moral distress. *Online Journal of Issues in Nursing, 15*(3), Manuscript 1. doi:10.3912/OJIN.Vol15No03Man01

Kagawa-Singer, M., & Blackhall, L.J. (2011). Negotiating cross-cultural issues at the end of life: "You got to go where he lives." In S.J. McPhee, M.A. Winker, M.W. Rabow, S.Z. Pantilat, & A.J. Markowitz (Eds.), *Care at the close of life: Evidence and experience* (pp. 417–428). New York, NY: McGraw-Hill.

Notes

Lachman, V.D. (2007). Moral courage in action: Case studies. *MEDSURG Nursing, 16,* 275–277.

McClendon, H., & Buckner, E.B. (2007). Distressing situations in the intensive care unit: A descriptive study of nurses' responses. *Dimensions of Critical Care Nursing, 26,* 199–206. doi:10.1097/01.DCC.0000286824.11861 .74

Murray, J.S. (2010). Moral courage in healthcare: Acting ethically even in the presence of risk. *Online Journal of Issues in Nursing, 15*(3), Manuscript 2. doi:10.3912/OJIN.Vol15No03Man02

Pask, E.J. (2003). Moral agency in nursing: Seeing value in the work and believing that I make a difference. *Nursing Ethics, 10,* 165–174. doi:10.1191/0969733003ne591oa

Pendry, P.S. (2007). Moral distress: Recognizing it to retain nurses. *Nursing Economics, 25,* 217–221.

Robinson, R. (2010). Registered nurses and moral distress. *Dimensions of Critical Care Nursing, 29,* 197–202. doi:10.1097/DCC.0b013e3181e6c344

Rushton, C.H. (2006). Defining and addressing moral distress: Tools for critical care nursing leaders. *AACN Advanced Critical Care, 17,* 161–168.

Unruh, J.A. (2010). Moral distress: A living nightmare. *Journal of Emergency Nursing, 36,* 253–255. doi:10.1016/j.jen.2010.03.01

Recommended Reading

Angelucci, P., & Carefoot, S. (2007). Working through moral anguish. *Nursing Management, 38*(9), 10, 12. doi:10.1097/01.NUMA.0000289282.72729.3a

Cavaliere, T.A., Daly, B., Dowling, D., & Montgomery, K. (2010). Moral distress in neonatal intensive care unit RNs. *Advances in Neonatal Care, 10,* 145–156. doi:10.1097/ANC.0b013e3181dd6c48

Cohen, J.S., & Erickson, J.M. (2006). Ethical dilemmas and moral distress in oncology nursing practice. *Clinical Journal of Oncology Nursing, 10,* 775–780. doi:10.1188/06.CJON.775-780

Coles, D. (2010). "Because we can…": Leadership responsibility and the moral distress dilemma. *Nursing Management, 41*(3), 26–30. doi:10.1097/01. NUMA.0000369495.69358.dc

Elpern, E.H., Covert, B., & Kleinpell, R. (2005). Moral distress of staff nurses in a medical intensive care unit. *American Journal of Critical Care, 14,* 523–530.

Ferrell, B.R. (2006). Understanding the moral distress of nurses witnessing medically futile care. *Oncology Nursing Forum, 33,* 922–930. doi:10.1188/06. ONF.922-930

Hamric, A.B., & Blackhall, L.J. (2007). Nurse-physician perspectives on the care of dying patients in intensive care units: Collaboration, moral distress, and ethical climate. *Critical Care Medicine, 35,* 422–429. doi:10.1097/01. CCM.0000254722.50608.2D

Jameton, A. (1984). *Nursing practice: The ethical issues.* Englewood Cliffs, NJ: Prentice Hall.

Notes

LaSala, C.A., & Bjarnason, D. (2010). Creating workplace environments that support moral courage. *Online Journal of Issues in Nursing, 15*(3), Manuscript 4. doi:10.3912/OJIN.Vol15No03Man04

McCue, C. (2011). Using the AACN framework to alleviate moral distress. *Online Journal of Issues in Nursing, 16*(1). doi:10.3912/OJIN. Vol16No01PPT02

Rogers, S., Babgi, A., & Gomez, C. (2008). Educational interventions in end-of-life care: Part I. An educational intervention responding to the moral distress of NICU nurses provided by an ethics consultation team. *Advances in Neonatal Care, 8,* 56–65. doi:10.1097/01.ANC.0000311017.02005.20

Shepard, A. (2010). Moral distress: A consequence of caring. *Clinical Journal of Oncology Nursing, 14,* 25–27. doi:10.1188/10.CJON.25-27

Internet Resources

American Association of Colleges of Nursing End-of-Life Nursing Education Consortium Core Curriculum: www.aacn.nche.edu/elnec/curriculum.htm

American Nurses Association Center for Ethics and Human Rights: www. nursingworld.org/MainMenuCategories/EthicsStandards.aspx

American Society for Bioethics and Humanities: www.asbh.org

Institute for Global Ethics: www.globalethics.org

Moral Courage Project: www.moralcourage.com

National Institutes of Health Bioethics Resources on the Web—Culture, Diversity and Health Disparities in Medicine: http://bioethics.od.nih. gov/culturalcomp.html

Oregon Health & Science University Center for Ethics in Health Care: www. ohsu.edu/ethics

Notes

DEPRESSION

Introduction

Depression in the healthy person may be a human response to sadness, grief and loss, disappointment, or feelings of failure. Nursing is an extremely emotional profession that taxes the nurse both physically and psychologically. Nurses follow patients and families along their journey of illness and, sometimes, grief and despair. In providing holistic care, nurses encourage patients and families to openly express their feelings and emotions; yet, paradoxically, this is often at the expense of suppressing their own grief (Boyle, 2000; Brown & Wood, 2009). The organizational stressors inherent in the profession of nursing today—high acuity, short staffing, the demands to do more with fewer resources—combined with the emotional demands of the work can predispose nurses to feelings of unrelieved stress, sadness, guilt, and worthlessness, thus increasing the risk of depressive symptoms (Lin, Probst, & Hsu, 2010; Weinberg & Creed, 2000). The traumatic states of compassion fatigue, vicarious traumatization, and secondary traumatic stress disorder all may influence nurses' risk for a mood disorder such as depression. The state of feeling "sad" is often referred to as *depression*; however, depression can range from acute, transient distress to a major psychiatric illness.

The major defining characteristics that differentiate normal and abnormal emotional responses to grief and loss are the *intensity, duration,* and *extent* to which the symptoms interfere with the nurse's ability to cope or function. The criteria for major depressive disorder as defined by the American Psychiatric Association (APA) are outlined in Figure 10. These criteria can be divided into *somatic* and *psychological* symptoms that are present almost every day during the same two-week period (Sivesind & Pairé, 2009). Somatic complaints include fatigue, insomnia, and an inability to think or concentrate. Psychological symptoms may range from depressed mood with crying spells, to diminished interest in usual activities, to feelings of hopelessness and helplessness. Other symptoms of depression include anxious or "empty" feelings, irritability, and restlessness. Anxiety often is closely linked with depressive mood. Some individuals with depression present with symptoms unrelated to feelings of sadness. Some individuals emphasize the somatic complaints (e.g., bodily aches and pains), whereas others may complain of irritability, outbursts of anger, or frustration (APA, 2000). People with depressive mood do not all experience the same symptoms. The severity, frequency, and duration of the symptoms will vary depending upon the individual and his or her particular illness. **At its most severe, depres-**

Figure 10. Criteria for Diagnosis of Depression in Medically Healthy Individuals

Somatic Symptoms
- Significant weight loss or gain
- Diminished ability to think or concentrate
- Psychomotor retardation or agitation
- Insomnia or hypersomnia
- Fatigue or loss of energy

Psychological Symptoms
- Depressed mood, crying spells
- Decreased self-esteem
- Feelings of helplessness and hopelessness
- Diminished interest or pleasure in usual activities (anhedonia)
- Recurrent thoughts of death or suicidal ideation

Note. Based on information from American Psychiatric Association, 2000.

From "Coping With Cancer: Patient and Family Issues" (p. 7), by D.M. Sivesind and S. Pairé in C.C. Burke (Ed.), *Psychosocial Dimensions of Oncology Nursing Care* (2nd ed.), 2009, Pittsburgh, PA: Oncology Nursing Society. Copyright 2009 by the Oncology Nursing Society. Reprinted with permission.

sion can lead to suicide. Therefore, depression needs to be readily identified and treated.

The important self-assessment criteria for the nurse to notice are whether these symptoms are a *change* from normal or baseline functioning and whether the symptoms continue unresolved for at least a *two-week* period. At least one of the symptoms must be (a) depressed mood or (b) loss of interest or pleasure (APA, 2000). Depression may range from mild to severe and is classified as major depression if the symptoms cause significant distress or impairment in the individual's social, occupational, and other important areas of functioning (APA, 2000). Symptoms must be unrelated to bereavement and must not be due to the side effects of medications, substance abuse, or a general medical condition (e.g., hypothyroidism) (APA, 2000).

Major depression can be biologic in nature. The physiologic mechanisms involved in depression are an imbalance of neurotransmitters (dopamine, norepinephrine, and serotonin) in the mood-sensitive regions of the brain (the limbic system, basal ganglia, and hypothalamus). The decrease in neurotransmitters, specifically serotonin, disrupts homeostatic mechanisms, thereby causing cognitive, behavioral, and systemic symptoms (Bush, 2009). People may have an increased risk of depression if they have a personal history of depression, depression in the family, or a history of post-traumatic stress, anxiety disorders, or substance abuse.

The rates and symptoms of depression differ between men and women. The lifetime risk of clinical depression is twice as high in women. Variables that increase a woman's risk for depression include gender differences in socialization, including ascribed roles, coping styles, and economic and social status (Bush, 2009; Kornstein & McEnany, 2000). Men may be less likely to report symptoms of depression because of fears related to the impact on job status or loss of health insurance benefits (Porche, 2005). Depression in men also may manifest differently than in women, with men displaying self-destructive behaviors such as using alcohol and drugs or engaging in reckless and risky behaviors. Suicide is either a symptom or a consequence of depression, and men are four times more likely to succeed at committing suicide (Porche,

Notes

Notes

2005). Male responses are more related to problem-solving coping strategies (action) than females, who respond with more emotion-focused coping styles. Gender differences may be due to socialization and biologic differences in the male and female brain (Johnson, 2009). Other variables that affect the incidence of depression include developmental life stage, cultural and socioeconomic factors, and social support (Bush, 2009).

Depression can be recurrent or chronic. It may cause disability, impairing people's ability to cope with daily life. It can be readily diagnosed and treated, yet many people deny or ignore the symptoms because of the stigma related to mental illness. There is a paucity of literature related to depression in the healthcare field and its impact on specific healthcare providers such as physicians and nurses. The culture of medicine often demands that healthcare providers suppress their own vulnerability and needs. The stigma with depression is a strong disincentive for obtaining adequate treatment (Middleton, 2008). Acknowledging feelings of sad mood, loss of interest in normal activities, feelings of guilt or low self-esteem, disturbed sleep or appetite, low energy, poor concentration, and feelings of hopelessness is the first step toward recognizing the need to reach out and seek appropriate help and treatment.

Interventions

Depression is a common but highly treatable disorder. The earlier that treatment is initiated, the more effective it is and the greater the likelihood that recurrence can be prevented. The stigma associated with mental illness causes many healthcare providers to deny the symptoms of depression or prevents them from seeking medical attention (Middleton, 2008). It is important for nurses to seek medical attention if they are suffering from (a) depressed mood or (b) absence of joy or pleasure in normal activities. Suicidal ideation and suicide attempts are common among depressed individuals, so the nurse must seek immediate medical attention if either is applicable.

REFLECTION

Depression Scale

Have any of the following symptoms been present nearly every day for at least two weeks?	Yes	No
1. Have you recently felt overwhelming sadness?		
2. Have you lost interest or pleasure in work activities or time with family/friends?		
3. Have you experienced a poor appetite or overeating, or a significant weight loss without dieting?		
4. Have you experienced insomnia or hypersomnia?		
5. Are you less talkative than usual or have you felt withdrawn?		
6. Do you find it difficult to be around other people?		
7. Have you lost interest or enjoyment in normally pleasurable activities?		
8. Is it hard to accept compliments when your work is praised or when you are shown attention?		
9. Do you have feelings of inadequacy or decreased feelings of self-esteem?		
10. Do you have feelings of worthlessness or guilt?		
11. Do you feel that you accomplish less at work or at home?		
12. Are you unable to think or concentrate, or are you feeling indecisive?		
13. Do you feel less able to cope with the responsibilities in your life?		
14. Do you have recurrent thoughts about death (not just fear of dying) or suicide ideation?		
15. Have you made a suicide attempt or a specific plan for committing suicide?		

Scoring of Depression Scale
Yes to question 1 or 2 or both—probable depressive illness/seek medical treatment*
Yes to question 14 or 15 or both—***urgently*** seek medical treatment
Yes to five or more questions—probable depressive illness/seek medical treatment*
No to questions 1, 2, 14, or 15—no serious depressive symptoms warranting immediate attention

*Medical conditions such as anemia and hypothyroidism and other physical ailments may mimic signs and symptoms of depression. Therefore, medical consultation should always include a thorough history and physical examination.
Note. Based on information from American Psychiatric Association, 2000; Klein & Wender, 2005.

Notes

Nurses can seek medical attention through their primary care physician or through a psychiatrist. If the nurse believes that a depressive disorder has developed, the first step is to reach out for help. Prior to treatment for depression, a thorough medical examination is advised. Some medical conditions, such as anemia or hypothyroidism, can cause the same symptoms as depression. If a medical condition is ruled out, then the primary care provider should perform a thorough psychological evaluation or refer the nurse to a mental health professional.

How will nurses know if the sadness they are experiencing warrants medical attention? Sadness is a normal part of the human experience. Many nurses are confronted with sadness throughout their work with patients who are traumatized, suffering from life-threatening illnesses, or facing death and dying. In people experiencing *sadness*, levels of dysfunction or distress are appropriate to the event (El-Mallakh, Wright, Breen, & Lippmann, 1996). If the nurse has a sudden onset of depressed mood related to the loss of a beloved patient, the symptoms may be appropriate for this life event. Dysfunction in social or occupational settings or a high level of subjective distress differentiates depression from transient sadness. It is chronic, unresolved sadness that places a person at high risk for depression. Other clues include a previous depressive illness or suicide attempt, a family history of a mood disorder, stressful life events, lack of social support, substance abuse, and concurrent chronic medical disease, pain, or disability (El-Mallakh et al., 1996). Symptoms of depression also may coexist with other major psychological disorders such as anxiety (see Chapter 9). Depression may be a result of chronic alcohol intake or alcohol and substance abuse. Substance abuse may be a form of self-medicating or a sign that the person is using alcohol or drugs as a coping mechanism against stress and sadness. If the nurse is experiencing any of the symptoms outlined, then it is prudent to seek medical attention.

The most common treatments for depression are psychotherapy and medication. Behavioral, cognitive, and interpersonal psychotherapies have shown moderate effectiveness for mild to moderate depression when used alone (Klein & Wender, 2005; Sharp, 2005). Interpersonal psychotherapy can provide people with the opportunity to explore emotions that may be influencing their mood, such as grief and loss, feelings of hopelessness or helplessness, or guilt. Cognitive-behavioral therapy approaches aim to help the person to recognize negative thought patterns that contribute to depression (e.g., "I am worthless") and help the person to reframe negative thinking and behaviors. People with mild depression may benefit from nonpharmacologic treatment models including exercise, social support, and cognitive-behavioral therapy tools along with psychotherapy (Sharp, 2005). Using relaxation techniques or guided imagery can help decrease the feelings of anxiety and tension that often accompany depression.

Pharmacotherapy plays a vital role in the treatment of major depression. Antidepressants work by normalizing naturally occurring brain chemicals such as serotonin and norepinephrine. Other antidepressants work on the neurotransmitter dopamine. The best therapy should be based on the presenting symptoms. The new selective serotonin reuptake inhibitors (SSRIs) are considered first-line therapy and are reported to be effective 50%–90% of the time (Sharp, 2005). This classification of drugs includes fluoxetine (Prozac®), citalopram (Celexa®), sertraline (Zoloft®), and several others. Serotonin-norepinephrine reuptake inhibitors, or SNRIs, are similar to SSRIs and include venlafaxine (Effexor®) and duloxetine (Cymbalta®). These drugs have become more popular than older classifications of antidepressants such as the tricyclics and monoamine oxidase inhibitors because of their profile of fewer side effects. Medication may take up to 4–8 weeks for an effective response and should be used for 6–12 months once remission is achieved to prevent relapse (Sharp, 2005). People with moderate to severe depression should be treated by a combination of both pharmacotherapy and psychotherapy.

Summary

Depression is a mood disorder characterized by unrelenting sadness and the loss of enjoyment in normal activities. Depression is biologic in nature and can be triggered by stressful life events. Risk factors include a personal history of depression, a family his-

Notes

tory of depression, a coexisting psychiatric illness, a chronic medical illness, lack of social support, and substance abuse. Nurses experiencing symptoms of depression should seek sound medical advice for assessment and treatment.

Case Study

Jenny was a young, vivacious 28-year-old nurse who worked on the burn unit of her local community hospital. She had worked there since graduation and had always found great reward in helping her patients survive from traumatic burns and be discharged home. Although she worked with highly traumatized patients, Jenny had always been able to cope effectively even when she felt extreme sadness if a beloved patient died from complications. Until recently, Jenny had felt inner peace about her life. She was happily married, she was healthy, and she had shown perseverance in reaching her personal goals to be a nurse. Jenny was surrounded by her loving husband and friends and socialized often with her colleagues.

Work had been especially difficult for the past nine months or so. Staffing had been cut, and nurses were working shorthanded and with patients with higher acuity. Jenny was also struggling in her personal life. Her mother had died unexpectedly of suicide just a year earlier, and Jenny was unsuccessfully trying to get pregnant. She blamed her inability to get pregnant on the grief she was experiencing over the loss of her mother and the stress at work. Over time, Jenny began to feel an overwhelming sense of sadness. At times she would find herself crying for what seemed like no reason at all. She expressed to her husband that she was always on the verge of tears.

At work, Jenny started to feel pressure from her added workload. It was hard for her to concentrate, and she felt sluggish and unable to accomplish as much as she usually did during her 12-hour shift. It would take her time after her shift was over to finish her charting before heading home. She found herself irritable and frustrated, often feeling angry toward her colleagues. Jenny even felt that she was avoiding talking to her patients about their distress because she felt she could not cope with their emotions flooding her own.

Each morning it was getting harder to go to work. Jenny wasn't sleeping well, but she was sleeping a lot. She would go to bed earlier at night because she lost interest in other activities, such as swimming, and even spending time with her husband felt exhausting. In the mornings she would swing her legs over the side of the bed and feel a heaviness she couldn't describe. Jenny was feeling like she was just "going through the motions." She was just so tired.

Discussion

Jenny has definite symptoms of depression, possibly triggered by the loss of her mother and her inability to achieve her goal of pregnancy. Her grief related to these losses was beginning to interfere with her personal, social, and occupational life. Jenny was not finding pleasure in her normal activities, including spending time with her husband. She was constantly feeling fatigued even though she spent a lot of time sleeping. Socially, Jenny found that she was having angry outbursts with the same colleagues whom she considered friends. Her work became difficult because she found it increasingly hard to concentrate. She was falling behind, thus making her stay late at night to finish her responsibilities.

Jenny couldn't pinpoint why she always felt she was on the verge of tears. Nor could she tolerate talking to her patients about their emotions without it overwhelming her own. These symptoms are a *change* from Jenny's usual vivacious personality. The symptoms began with the grief over her mother's death but intensified as the months passed. Nearly every day Jenny felt worse. In this case, Jenny would benefit from reaching out for help. She could begin by sharing her feelings with her husband or a trusted friend or colleague. A referral for a medical evaluation is in order to rule out any medical possibilities for her mood state, such as anemia or hypothyroidism, and to get a referral to a psychiatrist. Jenny's mother committed suicide, so this is a red flag for an increased risk of depression in her family. Jenny is suffering from moderate depression, which could worsen without treatment. Earlier treatment would be more effective and help to prevent a relapse. Both psychotherapy and pharmacotherapy are best suited in Jenny's case. She is showing somatic symptoms that would respond to medication, and psychotherapy would provide her with an avenue to gain insight into the grief she is suffering from her mother's suicide and how this could be affecting her mood and behaviors.

References

American Psychiatric Association. (2000). *Diagnostic and statistical manual of mental disorders* (4th ed., text rev.). Washington, DC: Author.

Boyle, D.A. (2000). Pathos in practice: Exploring the affective domain of oncology nursing. *Oncology Nursing Forum, 27,* 915–919.

Brown, C., & Wood, A. (2009). Oncology nurses' grief: A literature review. *Clinical Journal of Oncology Nursing, 13,* 625–627. doi:10.1188/09.CJON.625-627

Bush, N.J. (2009). Depression and anxiety. In C.C. Chernecky & K. Murphy-Ende (Eds.), *Acute care oncology nursing* (2nd ed., pp. 81–98). St. Louis, MO: Elsevier Saunders.

El-Mallakh, R.S., Wright, J.C., Breen, K.J., & Lippmann, S.B. (1996). Clues to depression in primary care practice. *Postgraduate Medicine, 100,* 85–88, 93–96. doi:10.3810/pgm.1996.07.9

Johnson, S.L. (2009). *Therapist's guide to posttraumatic stress disorder intervention.* San Diego, CA: Academic Press.

Klein, D.F., & Wender, P.H. (2005). *Understanding depression: A complete guide to its diagnosis and treatment.* New York, NY: Oxford University Press.

Kornstein, S.G., & McEnany, G. (2000). Enhancing pharmacologic effects in the treatment of depression in women. *Journal of Clinical Psychiatry, 61*(Suppl. 11), 18–27.

Lin, H.-S., Probst, J.C., & Hsu, Y.-C. (2010). Depression among female psychiatric nurses in southern Taiwan: Main and moderating effects of job stress, coping behaviour and social support. *Journal of Clinical Nursing, 19,* 2342–2354. doi:10.1111/j.1365-2702.2010.03216.x

Middleton, J.L. (2008). Today I'm grieving a physician suicide. *Annals of Family Medicine, 6,* 267–269. doi:10.1370/afm.840

Porche, D.J. (2005). Depression in men. *Journal for Nurse Practitioners, 1,* 138–139. doi:10.1016/j.nurpra.2005.09.013

Sharp, K. (2005). Depression: The essentials. *Clinical Journal of Oncology Nursing, 9,* 519–525. doi:10.1188/05.CJON.519-525

Sivesind, D.M., & Pairé, S. (2009). Coping with cancer: Patient and family issues. In C.C. Burke (Ed.), *Psychosocial dimensions of oncology nursing care* (2nd ed., pp. 1–28). Pittsburgh, PA: Oncology Nursing Society.

Weinberg, A., & Creed, F. (2000). Stress and psychiatric disorder in healthcare professionals and hospital staff. *Lancet, 355,* 533–537. doi:10.1016/S0140-6736(99)07366-3

Recommended Reading

Feskanich, D., Hastrup, J.L., Marshall, J.R., Colditz, G.A., Stampfer, M.J., Willett, W.C., & Kawachi, I. (2002). Stress and suicide in the Nurses' Health Study. *Journal of Epidemiology and Community Health, 56,* 95–98. doi:10.1136/jech.56.2.95

Van Fleet, S. (2006). Assessment and pharmacotherapy of depression. *Clinical Journal of Oncology Nursing, 10,* 158–161. doi:10.1188/06. CJON.158-161

Internet Resources

American Psychiatric Association: www.psych.org
American Psychological Association: www.apa.org
National Institute of Mental Health: www.nimh.nih.gov

ANXIETY

Introduction

Anxiety disorders are a common group of psychiatric disorders manifested by worry and distress. Symptoms of anxiety range from general feelings of nervousness to specific reactive behaviors such as panic. Most frequently, anxiety coexists with depression (see Chapter 8). Anxiety disorders are accompanied by objective disability and subjectively impaired quality of life (Stein, 2004). Although anxiety disorders may have an onset in childhood or adolescence and in many forms are interrelated, stressful events can trigger or compound an already existing anxiety disorder or uncover a new diagnosis. Anxiety disorders are medical conditions that respond effectively to appropriate treatment.

Anxiety is severe apprehension or worry about a real or perceived threat to personal safety. Anxiety may be a normal response to stressful life events, but it can become a pathologic condition if it persists and interferes with the person's ability to function. *Fear* is a normal affective response to a real threat, whereas *anxiety* is the affective response to a perceived threat or danger. Fear is the cognitive appraisal of a threat, and anxiety is the emotional response to that cognitive appraisal (Beck & Emery, 1985). Fear leads to the stress response of fight or flight; therefore, the physical symptoms of anxiety are associated with autonomic response, such as palpitations, shortness of breath, and feelings of being smothered. Anxiety associated with fear can cause the person to

Notes

be hypervigilant or emotionally paralyzed (Stein, 2004; Wolman, 1994). Symptoms of hypervigilance include scanning the environment, exaggerated startle response, difficulty concentrating or going blank, and difficulty falling asleep or staying asleep (American Psychiatric Association [APA], 2000).

The literature addressing anxiety in healthcare professionals is limited; therefore, the following is an overview of the types of anxiety that nurses may experience and the associated symptoms. Nurses who are at risk for being traumatized by their work or its environment may be at risk for anxiety. The inherent stressors in the empathic engagement with patients may trigger depression and associated anxiety if grief and loss are prolonged and unresolved.

Generalized anxiety disorder (GAD) is defined as excessive anxiety and worry (apprehensive expectation) related to activities of daily living (APA, 2000). The intensity, duration, and frequency of the anxiety are out of proportion to the actual likelihood or impact of the feared event, and the worry interferes with psychological and social functioning. Symptoms of anxiety can be related to apprehension, motor tension, autonomic hyperactivity, and vigilance (APA, 2000). In primary care, it is second only to depression as a major psychiatric disorder (Antai-Otong, 2003). For a diagnosis of GAD, the anxiety and worry are accompanied by at least three out of the following six symptoms and have lasted for most days over a period of at least six months: restlessness or feeling "on edge," fatigue, difficulty concentrating, irritability, muscle tension, and insomnia (APA, 2000). GAD may manifest in childhood or adolescence and affects more women than men (Marrs, 2006). A panic disorder may accompany or occur related to GAD.

A *panic attack* is a sudden onset of intense apprehension, fearfulness, or even terror associated with feelings of impending doom (APA, 2000). During a panic attack, the person will experience autonomic stimulation with symptoms such as chest pain, shortness of breath, and palpitations. It is not uncommon for individuals to feel like they are "going crazy" or losing control (APA, 2000). Other classifications of anxiety include specific or social phobias, agoraphobia, obsessive-compulsive disorder, acute stress disorder, and post-traumatic stress disorder. The definitions of these varied anxiety disorders are outlined in Table 2.

Table 2. Anxiety Disorders	
Disorder	**Definition**
Acute stress disorder	Symptoms similar to post-traumatic stress disorder but occurring immediately after the traumatic event
Agoraphobia	Avoidance of places or situations from which escape is perceived as difficult in the case of a panic attack
Generalized anxiety disorder	Characterized by six months of persistent and excessive anxiety and worry
Obsessive-compulsive disorder	Characterized by obsessions that cause anxiety and/or compulsions carried out to neutralize the anxiety
Panic attack	Sudden onset of intense apprehension, fearfulness, or terror associated with an impending sense of doom
Post-traumatic stress disorder	Reexperiencing of a traumatic event accompanied by increased arousal and avoidance of stimuli
Social phobia	Anxiety provoked by certain types of social or performance situations, leading to avoidance
Specific phobia	Anxiety provoked by exposure to a specific feared object or situation, leading to avoidance

Note. Based on information from American Psychiatric Association, 2000.

Notes

Wolman (1994) discussed the negative effects of anxiety on individuals and their worldview. An anxiety-ridden individual can be unhappy, worrisome, and pessimistic. Chronic anxiety can lead to a lasting and profound low self-esteem and feelings of helplessness. Anxiety can temporarily affect a person's intellectual function, especially memory and the ability to express oneself. Severe anxiety often produces feelings of inferiority, irritability, and anger toward oneself and others. Symptoms of anxiety can be immobilizing for the individual and can lead

Notes

to avoidance of feared objects or situations that provoke an anxious response.

Within the lexicon of nursing, anxiety may be exacerbated by an ability to control both workplace events and patient responses. The current healthcare environment is one characterized by accommodation. Fluctuating staffing models, evolving role expectations, and organizational restructuring place added demands on nurses to learn new skills, integrate new knowledge, embrace novel technology, and practice collaboratively with a changing work team (Greenglass & Burke, 2001). Inability to control or ameliorate the intensity or nature of the patient's or family's coping context further inhibits nurses' feelings of mastery. For staff with a preexisting anxiety disorder, limitations within this construct may stretch individual coping capacity.

Interventions

Anxiety interferes with family, cognitive, social, and occupational functioning. Individuals experiencing anxiety report a

---

REFLECTION

People enter nursing with their own individual styles, behaviors, and norms that are, in large part, dictated by their family. Anxiety is a coping response characterized by worry and distress. Ask yourself the following: Would I admit to being, or would others describe me as

- A worrier?
- Someone who gets stressed or frightened easily?
- A nervous type?
- Uneasy in situations where I do not know the routine or skill set?
- A ruminator, going over things repeatedly to reassure myself?
- Forgetful during times where multiple demands are placed on me?

If your general coping style is characterized by anxiety, anxiety will play a prominent part in your coping strategies at work and in your personal life. Problems may ensue when you feel overwhelmed and unable to perform as a result of the degree of anxiety manifested.

negative impact on quality of life, yet anxiety is a treatable medical disorder. The most effective treatments for anxiety disorders are psychotherapy and pharmacotherapy.

Psychotherapy for anxiety consists of behavioral and cognitive interventions. These therapies focus on principles of exposure to the perceived threat, desensitization to the perceived threat, and cognitive restructuring. Techniques include self-monitoring to increase awareness, countering catastrophic thoughts, and increasing exposure to and decreasing avoidance of anxiety-provoking stimuli (Stein, 2004). Psychoeducation may also play a role by dispelling myths associated with anxiety and educating people that anxiety is a medical condition that can be diagnosed and treated effectively (Stein, 2004), thus providing hope to those who are impaired by the disorder. Other psychotherapeutic interventions that may prove beneficial include relaxation techniques, biofeedback, and exercise (Marrs, 2006).

Pharmacotherapy plays an important role in the management of anxiety. Benzodiazepines are used for short-term treatment but have the disadvantages of cognitive impairment, oversedation, dependency, and problems with withdrawal. The selective serotonin reuptake inhibitors (SSRIs) have become the first-line treatment for a range of different anxiety disorders. SSRIs are reasonably effective and well tolerated, and an added benefit is that they are beneficial for both anxiety symptoms and comorbid mood disorders such as depression (see Chapter 8). Because of the chronicity of anxiety disorders, it is advised that medication be continued for one to two years. Psychotherapy along with pharmacotherapy may help individuals to maintain a treatment response (Stein, 2004). Second-line antidepressant drugs used for anxiety management are selective norepinephrine reuptake inhibitors (or SNRIs) or the older tricyclic antidepressants. Other classifications include beta-blockers and anticonvulsants (Marrs, 2006). Pharmacotherapy is best when aimed at the presenting symptoms and individual diagnosis and administered under the supervision of a trained physician or psychiatrist.

Notes

REFLECTION

Prominent Worries

The goal of this exercise is to delineate causes of anxiety that prevail in your life. By giving them names and identifying the situations in which they occur, you can plan interventions to decrease their intensity.

- Think about scenarios in your everyday life that cause you anxiety. They may be particular family circumstances, interpersonal relationships, skills, problem-solving capabilities, or anxiety-provoking situations in your work setting.
- Insert these worries within the outline of the person's head below. For those anxiety-provoking themes that concern you the most, write them in large letters, and for the smaller ones, write the words in smaller case. Hence, the size of the words should be relative to the size of the worry.
- Then take a few minutes to look over the graphic. Does anything surprise you? Pick out at least one of the themes where you can identify a solution to make the worry less prominent. Then consider an action plan to take and note it adjacent to where you cited the concern.

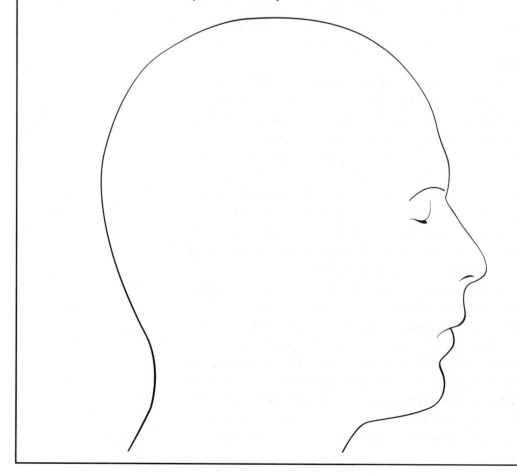

Summary

Anxiety is a disorder that manifests in excessive worry and distress. Anxiety can range from generalized anxiety to specific anxiety syndromes, such as acute stress disorder or post-traumatic stress disorder. Triggers for anxiety can exist in all settings and can negatively affect psychological, social, and occupational functioning. Anxiety is a medical disorder that is treatable with psychotherapy and pharmacotherapy. Individuals experiencing anxiety should also be assessed for associated mood disorders such as depression.

Case Study

John had been a critical care nurse for five years when he decided to return to graduate school to obtain his DNP. He enjoyed his job immensely and was mentored by a clinical nurse specialist (CNS) who served as his role model and advocate in encouraging him to pursue further studies. John always took advantage of educational activities so that he could learn more about his work with critically ill patients and their families. Going to graduate school seemed like the next step in his career ladder.

John did well his first year of school and was able to balance his work and family obligations with his school responsibilities. John's wife was also a nurse, so she was very supportive of his personal goals to advance his career. She was tolerant of his late-night studies and his time at school, which often decreased their own quality time together. John was excelling at his studies, and in the first year he found it exciting and easy to juggle all of his activities.

In his second year of graduate school, John started feeling increasingly anxious. He began to question the time he spent focusing on his own work instead of spending time with his wife. She had been inquiring about the possibility of starting a family soon after his graduation. This made John feel unsettled because he was still unsure of his future employment once he graduated. His work setting also was undergoing significant restructuring. Two critical care units were merging because of staffing constraints.

Notes

The medical and trauma intensive care units would soon be combined into one unit. John began having insomnia, poor eating habits, and a lack of routine exercise. He had always been able to integrate fitness into his life before going to school. However, now he felt he had limited time to spend on himself.

John began to feel nervous and unsure of his future. He would constantly ruminate about the fear of failing a test or doing poorly on the comprehensive examination necessary for graduation. He found himself irritable and often angry at his wife if she placed any demands on his time or attention. John also felt pressure from the demands of his job. There had been a high turnover of experienced staff in the past year, and as a senior nurse, he was always asked to precept and orient the newly hired. Although he had previously enjoyed such a commitment, he now felt that it took too much of his attention and energy and disrupted his concentration while working.

Recently, during the day shift, John was standing at the medicine station getting ready to do his patient rounds. It was a hectic day, with one patient imminently requiring intubation and another patient due for a complex dressing change. While John was organizing his thoughts, the critical care CNS approached him. She asked him about his interest in cochairing a unit-based taskforce with pharmacy the following week. John replied, "Sure," in his usual manner of helpfulness and support. As the CNS turned away, John began to feel faint. He experienced palpitations and shortness of breath. As he looked around, no one appeared to notice his sweaty palms and forehead. Suddenly, John felt an impending sense of doom. His chest tightened, and his head was swirling. John felt as though he could not do his job or balance his personal life any longer. He couldn't keep up with the stress. John felt like running, but in fact he stood there immobilized with overwhelming feelings of panic.

Discussion

Most likely, John was experiencing a panic attack. Although no real danger was at hand, John perceived this to be the case as building pressures consumed him. It is highly probably that John had been feeling anxious for more than a year while balancing his multiple responsibilities of family, work, and school. His lifestyle changes of little sleep, poor diet, and lack of routine exercise were contributing to his mounting stress levels.

Although no concrete threat to John's safety existed, he sensed a danger to his well-being. He abruptly began to doubt his ability to perform and succeed. His anxiety was also evident through his angry and resentful feelings toward his wife. John needed to recognize the symptoms of anxiety that he was experiencing and identify possible solutions. Initiating a routine exercise program to decrease his worry and learning relaxation techniques such as deep breathing and guided imagery could help reduce his emotional distress. John could ask his wife whether she had noticed changes in his behavior and solicit her help in brainstorming possible solutions to more effectively confront the anxiety he was feeling.

Continued evaluation of John's anxiety is warranted, as is the delineation of ongoing signs of comorbid depression. If self-care activities are not adequate to relieve John's anxious symptoms, then he should seek medical attention for appropriate treatment. Anxiety is an uncomfortable and distressing emotion and can further interfere with John's family, social, and occupational functioning.

References

American Psychiatric Association. (2000). *Diagnostic and statistical manual of mental disorders* (4th ed., text rev.). Washington, DC: Author.

Antai-Otong, D. (2003). Current treatment of generalized anxiety disorder. *Journal of Psychosocial Nursing and Mental Health Services, 41*(12), 20–29.

Beck, A.T., & Emery, G. (1985). *Anxiety disorders and phobias: A cognitive perspective.* New York, NY: Basic Books.

Greenglass, E.R., & Burke, R.J. (2001). Stress and the effects of hospital restructuring in nurses. *Canadian Journal of Nursing Research, 33,* 93–108.

Marrs, J.A. (2006). Stress, fears, and phobias: The impact of anxiety. *Clinical Journal of Oncology Nursing, 10,* 319–322. doi:10.1188/06.CJON.319-322

Stein, D.J. (Ed.). (2004). Introduction. In D.J. Stein (Ed.), *Clinical manual of anxiety disorders* (pp. 1–12). Washington, DC: American Psychiatric Publishing.

Wolman, B.B. (1994). Defining anxiety. In B.B. Wolman & G. Stricker (Eds.), *Anxiety and related disorders: A handbook* (pp. 3–10). New York, NY: Wiley.

Notes

Notes

Recommended Reading

Shear, M. (2003). Optimal treatment of anxiety disorders. *Patient Care, 37,* 18–32.

Starcevic, V. (2006). Anxiety states: A review of conceptual and treatment issues. *Current Opinion in Psychiatry, 19,* 79–83. doi:10.1097/01.yco .0000194146.81024.5a

Internet Resources

American Psychiatric Association: www.psych.org
American Psychological Association: www.apa.org
Anxiety Disorders Association of America: www.adaa.org
National Institute of Mental Health: www.nimh.nih.gov

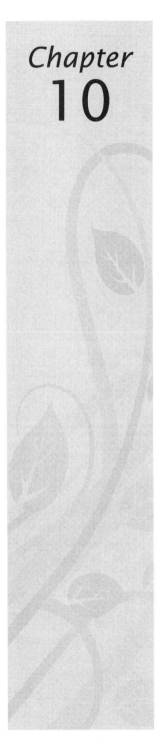

SELF–HEALING

Introduction

A central irony in nursing is that the majority of nurses perceive themselves as giving, caring people but find it hard to nurture themselves (Boyle, 2011). This is substantiated in reports of nurses' perceptions of their health. As many as 70% of nurses cite the acute and chronic effects of work-related stress as one of their top three health concerns (Collins, 2011). An international study of nurses from five countries reported that work-related stress was considerable and was associated with job turnover and decisions to terminate employment (Aiken, Clarke, & Sloane, 2002). Workplace stress awareness in nurses is growing, as evidenced by a slow but steady increase in organizational program offerings (McVicar, 2003; Stichler, 2009). Another indication of the recent predominance of nurse self-care issues is its escalating appearance in the nursing literature (Carroll-Johnson, 2010). One state nurses association has even written a position statement on the importance of nurses' self-care (New York State Nurses Association, 2005).

Self-care begins with healing. It requires a relentless pursuit of body, mind, and spirit balance. Self-care is grounded upon a healthy lifestyle with adequate nutrition, exercise, and sleep. Yet, if the nurse is wounded in mind and spirit, then physical and behavioral lifestyle changes may feel unattainable. Healing requires an active nurturance of the self. This workbook has addressed a variety of traumatic states that may contribute to nurses feeling overwhelmed and emotionally exhausted. Unresolved nurse grief may underlie many of the sequelae discussed. Nurses often remain resilient and demonstrate effective coping mechanisms. However, prolonged exposure to stressors in the absence of personal or professional resources to counter their deleterious effects can result in negative outcomes.

How does the nurse begin to identify the need for self-care? First and foremost, an acknowledgment of one's inherent risk for emotional, physical, and spiritual depletion caused by the demands of nursing must prevail. Much like how firefighters anticipate and prepare for threats to safety in their work settings, so must nurses ready themselves for risks to their well-being. Skovholt and Trotter-Mathison (2011) posed the query,

> How does the opera singer take care of the voice?
> The baseball pitcher, the arm?
> The woodcutter, the axe?
> The photographer, the eyes?
> The ballerina, the legs and feet?
> The counselor, therapist, health professional, teacher, the self? (p. xv)

For most nurses, self-care is a foreign topic. Nurses are frequently "other-directed" in their orientation, attending to the needs of others before—or instead of—their own. Scholar (2010) characterized many nurses as having "type E" personalities: doing **E**verything for **E**veryone **E**lse. This author also observed that when nurses are asked how they are doing, they usually respond, "I'm fine" (in other words, they **F**requently **I**gnore their **N**eeds and **E**motions).

The exercises in this workbook facilitate nurses' active choosing of strategies that foster wellness and resilience rather than avoidance and denial. Exhausted when saying yes, guilty when saying no, nurses who generally are emotionally attuned to the needs of others can benefit from interventions that augment professional vitality and minimize depleted caring. Nurses can prevent or minimize work-associated harm only when they anticipate and prepare for potential threats to their wellness.

Looking Within

Introspection is key to self-healing. Nurses need to contemplate for themselves, "What needs care and attention?" For example, is anger, guilt, or denial acting as a barrier to caring for oneself? Is a judgmental attitude fostering good/bad, right/wrong, or insensitive reactions to difficult patient and family scenarios? Stress perception is highly subjective (McVicar, 2003). Answers to your own personal inventory will help construct a meaningful wellness and self-healing action plan.

Although people are often cautioned to not bring their problems to work, actualizing this dictum is difficult. Nurses must consider to what degree personal issues are influencing their practice. How overwhelmed do they feel with the combination of home and work-related stressors? Are personal concerns and demands more problematic than their career-associated ones?

Notes

REFLECTION

A Personal Inventory of Stress

List your current stressors or concerns that have personal/home/family etiologies. Then rank the degree of their stressfulness.

Personal/Home/Family Stressors   *Not Stressful* 1 2 3 4 5 *Very Stressful*

1. _____   _____

2. _____   _____

3. _____   _____

4. _____   _____

5. _____   _____

Of the top three stressors identified, what action steps can you take to reduce their intensity?

Priority Personal/Home/Family Stressors   *Action Step*

1. _____   _____

2. _____   _____

3. _____   _____

Now, contemplate how you can integrate these actions into your lifestyle over the next week and month.

Notes

Another personal variable that requires reflection is that concerning professional boundaries. This refers to the limits or edges demarcating appropriate professional nurse behaviors from non-clinical or personal responses.

Boundary issues usually are indicative of some degree of over-involvement with patients or families. However, not all boundary crossings are boundary violations. Boundary violations often stem from unconscious needs and can have harmful end results. Nurses may displace or confuse their needs with the patient's (Sheets, 2001). When the care rendered exploits the patient or family and potentially puts them in jeopardy, then a violation has occurred. Self-disclosure, countertransference, or even secretive behavior may constitute boundary transgressions (Baca, 2011).

For example, an acute rehabilitation nurse alienated from her family and wanting close interpersonal connections may render advice and provide home visits outside of work for a patient she has grown fond of. Or, a single nurse mother with a teenager may ask if she could call a patient's wife for advice on how to discipline her son in the coming weeks. Asking oneself whether the nursing behavior in question is beyond usual nurse caring can help to determine if a boundary violation has occurred (McCaffrey, 1992). The recent explosion of social networking technology presents a plethora of opportunities for boundary crossings among nurses, patients, and families (Tariman, 2010). Boundary transgressions represent more than going the extra mile or having a simple discussion of what happened during your workday. They can have serious ethical and legal consequences, as the patient's right to privacy may be violated.

REFLECTION

Consider the following.
- How often have you extended yourself to a patient or family outside of the work setting? Ask yourself honestly, what prompted you to act this way?
- When have you discussed a patient or family scenario with non-coworkers? What was the context of the discussion? Why do you think this particular instance prompted you to talk about it outside of work?
- If you have been asked to befriend a patient or family member on Facebook or other social media forums, how have you responded?

Personal Attributes That Enhance Self-Healing

Resilience is a contemporary term often paralleled with *persever-ance*. It reflects effective coping in spite of adversity (Tugade & Fred-rickson, 2004). Resilience is typified by both skill and a personal phi-losophy to move beyond trauma and hardship. *Hardiness* refers to people's ability to maintain themselves below their stress threshold (McVicar, 2003). It is conceptualized as being one part of a cluster of factors that exemplify *innate resilience*. Other factors include adaptabil-ity, faith, optimism, patience, self-efficacy, self-esteem, tolerance, and having a sense of humor (Grafton, Gillespie, & Henderson, 2010).

Resilience is often thought of relative to patient coping. But nurses also possess this trait, and it can be transferred to the work setting. Although little research exists on this topic, a greater un-derstanding of how resilience can help nurses cope will assist edu-cators in their contemporary preparation of a highly skilled nurs-ing workforce (Zander, Hutton, & King, 2010).

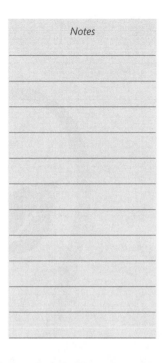

Notes

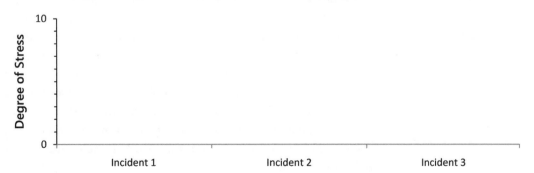

REFLECTION

Rearview Mirror Exercise

Reflect on your past and how you have manifested resilience. What helped sustain you in difficult times? Identify two or three critical experiences that you considered stressful. Draw a bar above Incident 1, Inci-dent 2, and Incident 3 relative to how stressful this occurrence was for you. Put the name of the incident below the bar (e.g., divorce, patient died, last child went off to college).

Degree of Stress — 10 ... 0

Incident 1   Incident 2   Incident 3

Now to the right of the bar, list what helped you get through this difficult experience. Consider how these coping strategies and/or supportive resources are currently evident in your life now or how you can retool them in your current situation.

Notes

Self-care is characterized by finding balance, maintaining a healthy lifestyle, setting limits, and connecting with others. Self-nurturance is treating oneself with gentleness and focusing on comfort, relaxation, and play (Saakvitne & Pearlman, 1996). Other descriptions of the aspects of self-care include
- Having self-compassion
- Experiencing compassion satisfaction
- Evolving from post-traumatic growth
- Establishing empathic equilibrium
- Maintaining conscious awareness of personal limits.

The work of nursing evolves within an environment laden with considerable emotional demands (Kravits, McAllister-Black, Grant, & Kirk, 2010). If nurses can identify their psychological needs, this is an important first step toward self-healing. This requires confronting denial, a major impediment to self-healing. When nurses disclaim their human response to the heart-wrenching challenges they face daily in practice, they negate their ability to heal from the inside out (Smith, 2009).

The concept of mindfulness represents insight into the experience of compassion fatigue, grief, and all the associated corollaries of intense nurse caring. *Mindfulness* can be defined as paying attention on purpose, in the present moment, and without judgment to the unfolding of experience moment to moment (Kabat-Zinn, 2003). One simple exercise includes "inhaling peaceful thoughts" and "exhaling your worries." Mindfulness-based stress reduction helps nurses in coping with the stress, emotional exhaustion, cynicism, and lack of a sense of accomplishment that can accompany burnout (Cohen-Katz, Wiley, Capuano, Baker, & Shapiro, 2004).

Healing the spirit is essential to living life to its fullest (Brown-Saltzman, 1994). For inner peace, a balance must exist between giving and receiving, and sadness and joy, that enables the nurse to continue to work with tenderness, empathy, and vulnerability. A key to managing sadness is identification of growth-enhancing versus self-destructive ways to stay mindful of one's emotional and behavioral responses to stress.

Self-care is a form of insulation against stress (Sherman, 2004). Exercising, getting adequate rest and sleep, and maintaining good nutrition are core competencies of self-care. Preventing compassion fatigue integrates these interventions and also may include challenging yourself to a higher level of spirituality and insight. Walk, meditate, and become one with nature. Practice what has been termed the *art of the possible,* meaning always do your best (Larson & Bush, 2006). Learning self-forgiveness and self-love is inherent in healing and preventing compassion fatigue. Being kind, gentle, and patient with yourself is one way in which you can effectively cope. Practice what you preach: You should treat yourself with the empathy and compassion that you share with patients and families. You can do this through reflective work, such as meditation, guided imagery, yoga, journaling, and other activities. Treat yourself to massage therapy or, if needed, interpersonal therapy. Creativity in the form of art, music, dance, and journaling can provide you with a "healing path" (Brown-Saltzman, 1997). Find support from relationships outside of the work setting. Identify something you look forward to each day.

Notes

REFLECTION

Undertake a self-care audit. Ask yourself, how and where do I spend my time? In the circle below to the left, allocate the percentage of your activities in your usual day. Be sure to designate a piece of the wedge for the appropriate amount of self-care time. Next to that wedge, write down what you do to care for yourself. Now in the circle below to the right, reconfigure your wedge to forcibly make more time for self-nurturance. Next to that wedge, write what new behaviors you can undertake.

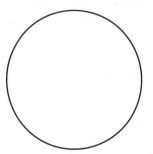

Current

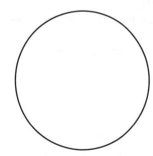

Future

Consider how much effort you are devoting to self-healing. Nurses dedicated to caregiving must develop a blueprint for health preservation. It is never too late to cultivate and apply self-directed care that nourishes and sustains all our resources—mental, physical, and spiritual (Smith, 2009).

(Continued on next page)

REFLECTION *(CONTINUED)*

Activity: Crafting Your Wellness Blueprint

Skovholt and Trotter-Mathison (2011) identified multiple personal domains that require nurturing, including the emotional, humorous, loving, nutritional, physical, playful, priority-setting, recreational, relaxing/stress-reducing, solitary, and spiritual selves. These represent a multifocal approach at evaluating all the components of one's life that require sustenance and rejuvenation.

In the following lists, circle three items within the 10 themes identified that appeal to you as possible new strategies to take better care of yourself. Consider options that you will enjoy rather than those you perceive as being extra work or adding more stress to your life. This is not an all-inclusive list. Space is provided in each section for you to add your own examples.

Nutritional

- Complete a diet journal.
- Attend a nutrition seminar.
- Sign up for Weight Watchers®.
- Read a book on health implications in disease prevention.
- Calculate your ideal weight based on age, gender, body surface area, or other nationally recognized guidelines.
- Read the labels on all grocery store purchases.
- Avoid eating at fast food restaurants.
- Read meal content information from restaurant menus.
- Avoid soda, fried foods, and high-sugar or sugary, processed foods.
- Avoid foods with highly saturated fatty meats.
- Minimize coffee consumption.
- Use smaller plates with smaller portions.
- Avoid desserts.

_____
_____
_____
_____
_____
_____
_____
_____
_____
_____

Physical

- Plan a graduated walking program.
- Walk with a colleague at lunch.
- Plan a short hike with a "fit" friend, and ask for help with establishing a program for yourself.
- Take the stairs at work rather than the elevator.
- Sign up to do a walk for a health awareness event.
- Ride your bike to the grocery store when you need a small amount of items.
- Walk rather than using the parking shuttle at work.
- Join an aerobics class that meets after work.
- Search the Internet for sites indicating caloric expenditures of physical activity.
- Engage in active playground time with young children.

_____
_____
_____
_____
_____
_____
_____
_____
_____
_____
_____
_____
_____

(Continued on next page)

REFLECTION *(CONTINUED)*

Stress-Reducing

- Start journaling.
- Sign up for a relaxation training course.
- Learn the art of meditation.
- Ask a friend to join you on a nature walk.
- Complete a sleep diary over a week's period of time.
- Keep a journal by your bed and describe your dreams.
- Take a nap when you are tired at home.
- Make an appointment for a massage.
- Sign up for a spa package with your best friend.
- Learn about music therapy.

_____

_____

_____

_____

_____

_____

_____

_____

_____

Emotional

- Practice saying no.
- Say no when you feel overwhelmed or have no energy.
- Don't apologize for knowing your limits.
- Ask for help.
- Consider the need for a counselor.
- Consider participating in a support group.
- Schedule lunch with a role model or mentor and ask for advice on a troublesome topic.
- Read books on a topic that you feel you need to have better skills with or knowledge about.
- Address losses in your personal life and consider how they are affecting your work.
- Journal your concerns.
- Prioritize the top three things you are worried about right now.
- Read up on the benefits of cognitive-behavioral therapy.

_____

_____

_____

Social

- Join a book club.
- Schedule dinner or coffee with a friend you have lost touch with.
- Plan time with friends whom you feel a special connection with.
- Write a letter to someone whom you hold close to your heart.
- Make an effort to expand your social network.
- Extend yourself to someone new to expand your social circle.
- Use close friends as a source of support; ask them how they have mastered difficulties.

_____

_____

_____

_____

Hobby/Play

- Go to the movies or rent a movie at least once a month.
- Schedule time to attend concerts, plays, or other events that bring you joy.
- Participate in sports that you enjoy.
- Read.
- Plan a trip or time away three to four times a year.
- Participate in an activity that makes you laugh.
- Spend time with a friend who has a good sense of humor.

_____

_____

_____

_____

_____

(Continued on next page)

REFLECTION *(CONTINUED)*

Spiritual

- Identify strategies to develop your spiritual life.
- Consider attending or participating in events that help you reflect on your inner strengths or establishing a relationship with a higher power.
- Pray.
- Read spiritual books or written commentaries on faith-based topics.
- Attend worship ceremonies.
- Incorporate generosity and thankfulness into your daily routine.

_____
_____
_____
_____
_____
_____
_____
_____
_____

Additive/Complementary

- Consider learning about, integrating into your life, or regularly using
  - Guided imagery
  - Therapeutic touch
  - Reiki
  - Massage
  - Acupuncture
  - Aromatherapy
  - Yoga
  - Herbal or vitamin therapy (with appropriate consultation).

_____
_____
_____
_____
_____
_____
_____
_____

Reduce Negative Lifestyle Choices

- Take a smoking cessation class.
- Speak with your primary healthcare provider about options to stop smoking.
- Track how much "social" drinking you do and when these episodes occur.
- Consider whether your alcohol consumption has increased, and if so, over what period of time.
- Ask whether the people around you have voiced concern about your alcohol use.
- Consider your use of sedatives and antianxiety medications and whether it has increased.
- Ask yourself if you are using other recreational forms of mood-altering substances.
- Record times of self-medication with substances and their corollary with stress.

_____
_____
_____
_____
_____

Partner/Family

- Make an appointment for a couple's massage.
- Establish a regularly scheduled "date night" for just you and your partner.
- Schedule routine partner/family events that foster connection, communication, and companionship.

_____
_____
_____
_____
_____
_____
_____
_____
_____
_____
_____

(Continued on next page)

REFLECTION *(CONTINUED)*

From this bank of 30 circled items, for the next two weeks, use at least one of these strategies daily. You may choose 14 different options or use one multiple times. Don't just hope you can find time to do them; schedule time for them. Much like you encourage your patients to establish a routine for taking their medications to ensure their optimum health, do the same for yourself.

Week 1	Activity	Time
Monday		
Tuesday		
Wednesday		
Thursday		
Friday		
Saturday		
Sunday		

Week 2	Activity	Time
Monday		
Tuesday		
Wednesday		
Thursday		
Friday		
Saturday		
Sunday		

In planning an improved approach to self-care, also remember the following.

- Do not immediately look for external solutions; rather, look within first. Pay attention to your inner life—your thoughts, feelings, and beliefs.
- Change takes time. Learning new skills and developing new patterns will not happen overnight. Take baby steps in actualizing your new approach.
- Consider strategies where you can partner with a colleague or friend. This often promotes more accountability, and

Notes

the camaraderie can enhance sustainability of the new activity.

- View your self-healing plan as establishing and validating your personal power, your own highly personalized prescription for health.

Considerations to Augment Self-Care at Work

The perimeter demarcating the personal from the professional life is gray at best. Many risk factors associated with substandard personal self-care can transcend to the work setting. The opposite is also true: negative work setting variables may influence coping and family dynamics at home.

Self-care embodies two complementary processes (Radziewicz, 2001). First, an awareness of personal limitations must be undertaken. Second, a commitment to engage in healing behav-

---

REFLECTION

The Poor Self-Care Deadly Dozen

A good example of the common blending of personal and professional life is represented in Skovholt and Trotter-Mathison's (2011) "Poor Self-Care Deadly Dozen." How many of the following characterize you?

___ 1. Toxic supervisor and colleague support

___ 2. Little fun (i.e., playfulness, humor, laughing) in life or work

___ 3. Only a fuzzy and unarticulated understanding of one's own needs

___ 4. No professional development process that turns experience into more competence and less anxiety

___ 5. Emotionally draining elements within one's personal life

___ 6. An inability to say no to unreasonable requests

___ 7. Vicarious traumatization that takes an accumulated toll

___ 8. Personal relationships characterized by one-way caring with the self consistently as the giver

___ 9. Constant perfectionism in work tasks

___ 10. Continual unresolved ambiguous professional losses

___ 11. A strong need to be needed

___ 12. Professional success defined solely by outward recognition or appreciation

Note. From *The Resilient Practitioner: Burnout Prevention and Self-Care Strategies for Counselors, Therapists, Teachers, and Health Professionals* (2nd ed., p. 257), by T.M. Skovholt and M. Trotter-Mathison, 2011, New York, NY: Routledge/Taylor & Francis Group. Copyright 2011 by Taylor & Francis Group. Adapted with permission.

iors must be embraced. Broadly, the psychological consequences of nursing emanate from witnessing health-related crises, exposure to interpersonal and intraprofessional conflict, and workload demands (Kravits et al., 2010). Specific to the work of nursing, multiple variables have been repeatedly noted to prompt feelings of emotional depletion and role inadequacy. Each of these will be briefly described followed by suggestions for workplace modifications to reduce their deleterious ramifications.

Inexperience

Novice nurses are especially vulnerable to being overwhelmed. Attempting to juggle the complex needs of multiple patients, they often function on survival mode, striving to get the basics done within a confined time frame. New nurses lack a critical-thinking skill set, so their focus is limited and their energy is targeted on recalling textbook-based facts. The curriculum-driven ideal of nurse perfectionism sets the stage for unrealistic expectations. In the absence of a seasoned mentor or guide to foster adaptability and role immersion, new nurses may continue to struggle with their unfolding practice and ultimately label themselves as inadequate or marginal at best.

The nursing literature is replete with commentary and models attesting to the benefits of preceptors for novice nurses. Although a definitive quantification of program type and length and profile of ideal mentor characteristics remains in question, what is not lacking is the recognition that new staff require formal support in adapting to their early months and years as a nurse (Hatler, Stoffers, Kelly, Redding, & Carr, 2011). Nursing work is just too complex and demanding to assume it can be actualized without coaching following licensure attainment. Hence, in addition to formal role enculturation offerings, other options to support inexperienced nurses in practice may include the following.

- Use a Likert scale–based stress thermometer to help new staff rank their work setting anxiety. This augments recognition and depiction of stress prompts and can be used to chronicle patterns of stress over time.
- Establish a "lunch buddies" program where well-respected seasoned nurses are teamed with new staff. The focus of discussion

Notes

at lunch should be coping, hardiness, resilience, and the identification of personal strategies and professional suggestions to enhance stress reduction and wellness. This type of intervention can be considered a form of clinical supervision similar to psychology and social work models (Mackereth, White, Cawthorn, & Lynch, 2005).

- Carry out patient and family focus groups to help identify how needs were met. This can be very beneficial for novice nurses to evaluate outcomes and, if necessary, change future interventions.

- Provide a forum or patient rounds with other team members such as the chaplain, social worker, or psychiatric liaison clinical nurse specialist. This will provide new nurses with an avenue to expand their psychosocial awareness and can also provide an opportunity for expression of personal anxieties or concerns.

Workload Challenge

Nursing is a complex profession characterized by myriad stressors. These stressors produce demands on the nurse that are both generic and specialty-specific in nature. Demands common to all of nursing are maintaining a sense of hypervigilance while monitoring patient status, responding to the changing acuity of patients, practicing in the context of staffing inadequacies, juggling care of multiple patients concurrently, and adapting to new technology and treatment approaches. Nurses also must interact with patients and family members with a wide range of personality types and coping styles and witness patient and family despondency and suffering. Additional requirements of the role are responding to organizational requirements and constraints (i.e., documentation), collaborating with a fluctuating group of team members, experiencing communication and boundary issues with team members, advocating for or giving voice to patient concerns, feeling tense, anxious, or frustrated over ethical dilemmas, and feeling responsible for patients' safety and for anticipating their needs or considering preventive care interventions. Nurses often feel emotionally and physically drained with work challenges (including the demands of shift work) and strained with time demands. The American Association of Critical-Care Nurses (2005) has developed a series of standards for the workplace to promote environments that support and foster excellence in patient care. These standards recognize the vital importance of issues such as staffing and the meaningful recognition of nurses that deter the stressors mentioned (see Chapter 1).

Specialty-specific nurse stressors are those that emanate from the needs of a unique patient cohort and their associated medical management. For critical care, emergency department, and oncology specialties, nursing the dying patient has its own set of competencies and related stressors. Perioperative nurses must reduce distress in tandem with altered patient consciousness. Nephrology nurses must be expert in nutritional interventions and fostering adherence. Pediatric nurses require adaptability and versatility in working with children of varying developmental stages and their families. Gerontology nurses must be skilled in managing syndromes unique to older patients (i.e., falls, incontinence, cognitive alterations). Hence, the workplace context is one often characterized by escalated tension and ongoing demand, with nurses feeling that many of these challenges remain out of their control.

The New York State Nurses Association (2005) position statement advocates for work environments that are healing and nurturing for both staff and patients through improved communication, collaboration, empowerment, and accountability. They also recommend the use of debriefing interventions and support groups for nurses to address the emotional strain inherent within nursing. Another way of depicting this ideal work culture for nurses is to foster a practice environment known for its reciprocity of caring (Cohen, Brown-Saltzman, & Shirk, 2001). This means that behaviors among coworkers reflect acknowledgment of the caring that nurses extend to their patients and that they get back what they give to others. A caring milieu is palpable amongst the team to the same extent that it is evidenced with patients and families.

Overeating, smoking, and substance abuse are examples of ineffective coping behaviors employed by nurses (Kravits et al., 2010). Programs that address weight control, smoking cessation,

Notes

Notes

and reduction of mood-altering behaviors, offered in close proximity to the work setting, are beneficial. On-site education and intervention programs (such as a fitness club/gym, walking program, or personal stress management planning) to increase physical activity and offer dietary counseling can foster overall health promotion (Conn, Hafdahl, Cooper, Brown, & Lusk, 2009; Flannery, Resnick, Galik, & Lipscomb, 2011).

Because of the diversity of nurses in terms of style and need, a menu approach offering workplace wellness programs to reduce stress is ideal (Boyle, 2011). Complementary approaches that provide an outlet for stress and promote reflection and self-care are outlined in Figure 11.

Figure 11. Complementary Approaches to Workplace Interventions

- Acupuncture
- Aerobics
- Aromatherapy
- Art therapy
- Humor therapy
- Massage
- Meditation
- Mindfulness training
- Music therapy
- Pet therapy
- Relaxation
- Spiritual reflection groups
- Yoga

REFLECTION

Pick two items from Figure 11 that you feel would be helpful to initiate in your work setting. Then, identify the resource person(s) in administration whom you could approach with the idea and obtain approval.

Item:

_____

_____

Resource Person:

_____

_____

Lack of Team Cohesion

Interdisciplinary conflict may cause more stress for staff than interactions with patients and families (Mulder & Gregory, 2000). Conflict may ensue because of boundary issues and role overlap among disciplines. Colleagues may disagree on the goals of care for patients. Various members of the nursing team may focus on differing priorities (i.e., nurse managers are concerned about cost versus the nursing assistant taking breaks). Interventions that combat team conflict and stress should be carried out to promote teamwork and cohesion.

Management needs to acknowledge the stressful nature of nursing work and offer organizational support to counter workplace stress (Sherman, 2004). A culture of caring must be fostered that transmits management's recognition of the value of staff efforts and psychosocial needs (White, 2006). Longo's (2011) research addressed staff nurse perceptions of the creation of a caring environment in the work setting. Three subcategories of nurse caring behaviors specific to interactions with peers and coworkers included caring through helping and supporting, caring through appreciating, and acknowledging unappreciated caring.

Tributes to staff can take place in different forums. Team and peer recognition is the acknowledgment of a job well done by all team members contributing to common goals and outcomes. "Pat on the Back" is formal appreciation of the positive attributes of colleagues posted visibly on unit bulletin boards or in other mediums such as Web pages or newsletters. "Stretching encouragement muscles" (Carroll-Johnson, 2010) involves open acknowledgment of the dilemmas that colleagues face by extending words of support and appreciation for a job well done and recognizing all team members.

Using a shared governance model is a form of community building in the workplace (Medland, Howard-Ruben, & Whitaker, 2004). Within shared governance, all team members can address issues such as recruitment needs, staff retention, establishment of a rewards council, and bereavement programs. Important to the success of shared governance is staff encouragement to design programmatic needs as assessed by all team members

Notes

involved in patient care. Lastly, the psychosocial and self-care implications of specialty work should be developed and discussed upfront as part of shared governance and accountability (Lavoie-Tremblay et al., 2005).

Deficiency in Communication Skills

Basic nursing education uniformly fails to address the necessary communication skills required of nurses in their rendering of patient care. Learning is targeted on physical problems to the exclusion of a parallel focus on how humans adapt to health crises and the supportive counsel required by nurses that augments patient healing and recovery. However, novel approaches to enhancing students' skills in communication and the provision of emotional support have embraced the provision of seminars in undergraduate education that foster interdisciplinary learning (Chan, Mok, Po-ying, & Man-chun, 2009). This team approach to learning in basic education (versus a uniprofessional approach) is ideal, as it sets the stage for a team interface, which will be the foundation of nursing practice following graduation. Nurses in practice require continuing education, skill building, and opportunities to address the affective domain of their practice to bridge the evident knowledge and competency gap. Numerous options can be employed.

Formal education programs can address core principles in communication skill building integrating both didactic and interactive learning approaches. The delineation of evidence-based aspects of therapeutic communication within the psychosocial domain of nursing practice can enhance the reframing of nurse interactions from one that is critical and often characterized by negative self-talk (i.e., "I'm just not good at talking with patients") to one perceived as therapeutic (i.e., "I did a good job supporting Mr. Smith's children during that difficult encounter") (Collins, 2011). A review of verbal and nonverbal aspects of communication can also foster nurses' recognition of how to be a healing presence with patients, an important component of supportive care (McDonough-Means, Kreitzer, & Bell, 2004). Programs can be offered at basic and advanced levels. Other components of formal communication skill enhancement include courses in stress/

conflict reduction and coping with compassion fatigue (Kravits et al., 2010; Potter et al., 2010; Walton & Alvarez, 2010). Some office practices employ counselors to lead "brown bag" lunches once a month where staff discuss patient interactions or request formal mini-lectures on a host of topics. Additionally, on-site support groups and off-site retreats for staff have been used to address staff coping needs and enhance team building. Novel interventions such as the Tea for the Soul program led by pastoral care staff to render nurse support have been effective (see Chapter 5). Increasing popularity of the Schwartz Center Rounds (www.theschwartzcenter.org) has been cited in the literature. These rounds frequently focus on loss, end-of-life issues, and bereavement responses by staff (Lally, 2005).

Debriefing is an example of a reflective process that values knowledge embedded in experience. It fosters an experiential review of performance that promotes active learning. Debriefing clarifies what happened, what actions were effective and problematic, and what could be done differently to improve care in the future (Raphael & Wooding, 2004). It should not unfold within a dominant paradigm of blame or negativity. Rather, accomplishments, successes, and best practices require parallel attention. This examination and questioning allows nurses and their colleagues to contextualize and make sense of unusual or emotionally laden scenarios in practice (Wakefield, 2000). Debriefing is psychoeducational in nature. It can promote cognitive restructuring and can be a transforming experience. The ideal timing of debriefing has historically been proposed to occur within 24–48 hours following the event. The leader of debriefing reviews should have expertise in the clinical area, be skilled in group dynamics, and have the respect of the team engaged in the exercise. Again, the ultimate goal is growth, transcendence, and improved care delivery.

Exposure to Loss and Death

True compassion requires nurses to share the suffering, walk with patients and families, and bear witness to life's closure (Radziewicz, 2001). A side effect of this domain of nursing care is frequently the predominance of hidden sorrow and disenfran-

Notes

chised grief. Nurses struggle with the dichotomy of intimacy and restraints, which in and of itself is a major stress (Dowling, 2008; Wakefield, 2000). The stressful nature of nursing the dying does not discriminate by geographic boundaries. A multinational study of workplace stressors in Japan, Thailand, South Korea, and the United States identified that nursing dying patients represented the highest of all potential stressors for nurses (Lambert et al., 2004).

Even when the occurrence of death is not common, the experience can have lasting effects on the psyche of those who witness the loss. Foresman-Capuzzi (2007) described this phenomenon as a "low volume, high stress encounter" (p. 505), as in the unexpected death of a child in the emergency department. What is important for the nurse is to be able to identify those variables that increase the risk of intense grief and loss related to death and dying. Knowing these variables can act as personal alerts for the nurse and include situations such as when the nurse has an established relationship with the patient, when multiple concurrent deaths are likely to occur in the specialty practice, when there is ineffective symptom management causing distress in the patient, and when caring for a patient case that has ethical quandaries related to communication deficiencies.

A number of potential workplace interventions exist to address the emotional labor of nurses when confronted with death and dying. Wenzel, Shaha, Klimmek, and Krumm (2011) delineated six clusters of recommendations to support nurses:
- Creating time and space for staff self-care
- Counseling or communicating with others who understand
- End-of-life issues and hospice or palliative care initiatives
- Quality time with patients and families
- Acknowledgment and reinforcement of nurses' special efforts
- Work structures, work processes, and organization.
All of these domains require work setting innovation and new learning.

Education related to death and dying is extremely important for nurses working in specialty areas where death may be more common such as oncology, critical care, and palliative care. Education could be in the form of mandatory classes, for example, the End-of-Life Nursing Education Consortium or in the form of grief workshops or retreats offered on a regular basis.

Brosche (2007) discussed the importance of establishing a grief team within each healthcare system to support staff grief. "When resources are properly utilized and healthcare providers feel that it is acceptable to grieve, they will be able to grieve in their own manner and at their own time, knowing that they are cared for and supported by the healthcare system" (p. 22). Interventions for grief support can be institutional or unit based. On-site counseling should be made available to team members through psychologist intervention and the support of chaplain and social services. The negative stigma associated with counseling can be addressed by normalizing reactions that evolve on a repeated basis (Mackereth et al., 2005). Actual bereavement protocols can be instituted, such as those found in emergency departments, intensive care, and perinatal services (Brosche, 2007; Foresman-Capuzzi, 2007). An ethics committee should also be a part of the bereavement team if the death has included ethical concerns.

Unit-based interventions can include the initiation of a grieving cart (see Chapter 5) and encouragement of behaviors that allow nurses to express their feelings. This may include prayer during or after the death, keeping a diary or journal that includes reminiscing about the loss, or carrying out an actual remembrance ceremony or memorial service. These interventions provide nurses with the opportunity to share both positive and negative feelings related to the death and, in turn, prevent the nurse from becoming a secondary victim (Foresman-Capuzzi, 2007) through vicarious traumatization. Bereavement or sympathy cards signed by the staff should be a form of follow-up for both the nurses and the family, and attendance at funeral or memorial services should be an option.

Mindfulness training for staff can also prove beneficial. Mindfulness consists of controlled breathing and emptying the mind by being in the present (Collins, 2011). This technique can be carried out prior to each shift by bringing the staff together for what has been called a "centering" activity—a moment of mindfulness that aids the staff to focus on being present for patients

Notes

Notes

and families (Collins, 2011). Centering also can be in the form of silent prayer, a relaxation technique, or reviewing the goals for patient care that shift.

Summary

Nurses are paramount in providing and sustaining the human connection between the patient and family and the rest of the healthcare team (Hinds, 2011). Nurses are heart-driven and thus are at risk for experiencing emotional challenges that emanate from the close proximity they have to those who are suffering. An active rather than passive approach to caring for the self has historically been understated and undervalued within nursing. However, it is a much-needed behavioral competency in today's health care. The New York State Nurses Association (2005) encouraged further research to identify the relationship between nurses who practice self-care and the outcomes for their patients. Douglas (2010) poignantly stated:

> Intuitively we know that when someone who is delivering care is out of balance, emotionally spent, or has lost their capacity for compassion, this is not a good thing. But how often does this occur, how well is it recognized, how often does it change our staffing or assignments, and do we take actions to help the individual get back in balance? (p. 415)

Nursing resourcefulness requires considerable scrutiny and, most certainly, further investigation. At best, ongoing evaluation of staff needs for those who render care is required (Qaseem, Shea, Connor, & Casarett, 2007). Assuming responsibility for self-healing is best regarded as a multistep process. First must be the recognition and acceptance of the nurse's inherent risk. Second is the individualized planning of a self-care blueprint that is customized to one's needs. Third, the strategies often require modification to make the plan practical and realistic, and thus sustainable. Throughout this process, nurses must maintain a consistent dose of egocentricity that validates their needs, worth, and the necessary consumption of personal and professional capital to enable them to persevere.

Implied within the delineation of action steps and interventions to foster self-care is an emphasis on strengthening nurses' capabilities and inner resources. Focusing on the positive, such as generating hardiness, helps reframe the context of nursing from one of stress and vulnerability to one of resilience and effective engagement. Bauer-Wu (2005) identified characteristics of nurse "thrivers," those capable of flourishing despite constant exposure to work-related stressors. She delineated the following prescription to be a nurse thriver.

- Be self-sufficient and have a "can do" attitude.
- Do fulfilling and enjoyable activities.
- Have at least one supportive and trusted relationship.
- Express a full range of emotions.
- Find meaning in your work every day.
- Partner with patients and colleagues.
- Engage often in stress-reducing activities.
- Have a sense of spiritual connection, including connection with nature.
- Be flexible and willing to try new things and to think outside the box.

Foundational to nursing is the struggle between altruism and self-preservation within the ubiquitous human drama of illness. How does one nurse, patient after patient, tragedy after tragedy? This paradigm of layered suffering deserves urgent attention (Purnell & Mead, 2007). Restoration, a constant investment in one's renewal process, is necessary for growth (Skovholt & Trotter-Mathison, 2011). Attempts at self-caring and interventions for self-healing foster an abiding resilience required to walk with patients through their health crises.

The intent of this workbook has been to give a newfound voice to the inner affective challenges of being a nurse. No other healthcare professional has inherent in the job description the expectations for biopsychosocial competency in the context of illness and tragedy coupled with the unique human connectivity born of presence, constancy, and advocacy. Practicing within the epicenter of illness and loss, nurses must ensure that their well-being is

Notes

Notes

cultivated with the same rigor, intensity, and expertise extended to those they nurse. As Cohen et al. (2001) noted, nurses truly embrace the value of compassionate care when they treat themselves compassionately. As a highly proficient yet vulnerable collective of nurturers, we must remember to heal ourselves.

References

Aiken, L.H., Clarke, S.P., & Sloane, D.M. (2002). Hospital staffing, organization and quality of care: Cross-national findings. *Nursing Outlook, 50,* 187–194. doi:10.1067/mno.2002.126696

American Association of Critical-Care Nurses. (2005). *AACN standards for establishing and sustaining healthy work environments: A journey to excellence.* Retrieved from http://www.aacn.org/WD/HWE/Docs/HWEStandards.pdf

Baca, M. (2011). Professional boundaries and dual relationships in clinical practice. *Journal for Nurse Practitioners, 7,* 195–200. doi:10.1016/j.nurpra.2010.10.003

Bauer-Wu, S. (2005). Seeds of hope, blossoms of meaning. *Oncology Nursing Forum, 32,* 927–933. doi:10.1188/05.ONF.927-933

Boyle, D.A. (2011). Countering compassion fatigue: A requisite nursing agenda. *Online Journal of Issues in Nursing, 16*(1), Manuscript 2. doi:10.3912/OJIN.Vol16No01Man02

Brosche, T.A. (2007). A grief team within a healthcare system. *Dimensions of Critical Care Nursing, 26,* 21–28. doi:10.1097/00003465-200701000-00007

Brown-Saltzman, K.A. (1994). Tending the spirit. *Oncology Nursing Forum, 21,* 1001–1006.

Brown-Saltzman, K. (1997). Replenishing the spirit by meditative prayer and guided imagery. *Seminars in Oncology Nursing, 13,* 255–259.

Carroll-Johnson, R.M. (2010). With a little help from our friends [Editorial]. *Oncology Nursing Forum, 37,* 657. doi:10.1188/10.ONF.657

Chan, E.A., Mok, E., Po-ying, A.H., & Man-chun, J.H. (2009). The use of interdisciplinary seminars for the development of caring dispositions in nursing and social work students. *Journal of Advanced Nursing, 65,* 2658–2667. doi:10.1111/j.1365-2648.2009.05121.x

Cohen, M.Z., Brown-Saltzman, K., & Shirk, M.J. (2001). Taking time for support. *Oncology Nursing Forum, 28,* 25–27.

Cohen-Katz, J., Wiley, S.D., Capuano, T., Baker, D.M., & Shapiro, S. (2004). The effects of mindfulness-based stress reduction on nurse stress and burnout: A quantitative and qualitative study. *Holistic Nursing Practice, 18,* 302–308.

Collins, S.B. (2011). From "distress" to "de-stress" with stress management. Retrieved from http://ce.nurse.com/ce424

Conn, V.S., Hafdahl, A.R., Cooper, P.S., Brown, L.M., & Lusk, S.L. (2009). Meta-analysis of workplace physical activity interventions. *American Journal of Preventive Medicine, 37,* 330–339. doi:10.1016/j.amepre.2009.06.008

Douglas, K. (2010). When caring stops, staffing really doesn't matter. *Nursing Economics, 28,* 415–419.

Dowling, M. (2008). The meaning of nurse–patient intimacy in oncology care settings: From the nurse and patient perspective. *European Journal of Oncology Nursing, 12,* 319–328. doi:10.1016/j.ejon.2008.04.006

Flannery, K., Resnick, B., Galik, E., & Lipscomb, J. (2011). Physical activity and diet-focused worksite health promotion for direct care workers. *Journal of Nursing Administration, 41,* 245–247. doi:10.1097/NNA.0b013e31821c464d

Foresman-Capuzzi, J. (2007). Grief telling: Death of a child in the emergency department. *Journal of Emergency Nursing, 33,* 505–508. doi:10.1016/j.jen.2007.06.011

Grafton, E., Gillespie, B., & Henderson, S. (2010). Resilience: The power within. *Oncology Nursing Forum, 37,* 698–705. doi:10.1188/10.ONF.698-705

Hatler, C., Stoffers, P., Kelly, L., Redding, K., & Carr, L.L. (2011). Work unit transformation to welcome new graduate nurses: Using nurses' wisdom. *Nursing Economics, 29,* 88–93.

Hinds, P.S. (2011). "Will you be there for me?" The human connection in oncology nursing care [Editorial]. *Cancer Nursing, 34,* 87–88. doi:10.1097/NCC.0b013e3182071b6a

Kabat-Zinn, J. (2003). Mindfulness-based intervention in context: Past, present and future. *Clinical Psychology: Science and Practice, 10,* 144–156. doi:10.1093/clipsy.bpg016

Kravits, K., McAllister-Black, R., Grant, M., & Kirk, C. (2010). Self-care strategies for nurses: A psycho-educational intervention for stress reduction and the prevention of burnout. *Applied Nursing Research, 23,* 130–138. doi:10.1016/j.apnr.2008.08.002

Lally, R.M. (2005). Oncology nurses share their experiences with bereavement and self-care. *ONS News, 20*(10), 4–5, 11.

Lambert, V.A., Lambert, C.E., Itano, J., Inouye, J., Kim, S., Kuniviktikul, W., … Ito, M. (2004). Cross-cultural comparison of workplace stressors, ways of coping and demographic characteristics as predictors of physical and mental health among hospital nurses in Japan, Thailand, South Korea and the USA (Hawaii). *International Journal of Nursing Studies, 41,* 671–684. doi:10.1016/j.ijnurstu.2004.02.003

Larson, D.G., & Bush, N.J. (2006). Stress management for oncology nurses: Finding a healing balance. In R.M. Carroll-Johnson, L.M. Gorman, & N.J. Bush (Eds.), *Psychosocial nursing care along the cancer continuum* (2nd ed., pp. 587–601). Pittsburgh, PA: Oncology Nursing Society.

Lavoie-Tremblay, M., Bourbonnais, R., Viens, C., Vézina, M., Durand, P.J., & Rochette, L. (2005). Improving the psychosocial work environment. *Journal of Advanced Nursing, 49,* 655–664. doi:10.1111/j.1365-2648.2004.03339.x

Longo, J. (2011). Acts of caring: Nurses caring for nurses. *Holistic Nursing Practice, 25,* 8–16. doi:10.1097/HNP.0b013e3181fe2627

Mackereth, P.A., White, K., Cawthorn, A., & Lynch, B. (2005). Improving stressful working lives: Complementary therapies, counselling and clinical supervision for staff. *European Journal of Oncology Nursing, 9,* 147–154. doi:10.1016/j.ejon.2004.04.006

Notes

McCaffrey, D. (1992). Cancer nurse stress: A paradigm with relevance to investigational biotherapy. In R. Carroll-Johnson (Ed.), *Biotherapy of cancer* (pp. 22–27). Pittsburgh, PA: Oncology Nursing Society.

McDonough-Means, S.I., Kreitzer, M.J., & Bell, I.R. (2004). Fostering a healing presence and investigating its mediators. *Journal of Alternative and Complementary Medicine, 10*(Suppl. 1), S25–S41. doi:10.1089/acm.2004.10.S-25

McVicar, A. (2003). Workplace stress in nursing: A literature review. *Journal of Advanced Nursing, 44*, 633–642. doi:10.1046/j.0309-2402.2003.02853.x

Medland, J., Howard-Ruben., J., & Whitaker, E. (2004). Fostering psychosocial wellness in oncology nurses: Addressing burnout and social support in the workplace. *Oncology Nursing Forum, 31*, 47–54. doi:10.1188/04.ONF.47-54

Mulder, J., & Gregory, D. (2000). Transforming experience into wisdom: Healing amidst suffering. *Journal of Palliative Care, 16*(2), 25–29.

New York State Nurses Association. (2005). Position statement: Self care. Retrieved from http://www.nysna.org/practice/positions/position22.htm

Potter, P., Deshields, T., Divanbeigi, J., Berger, J., Cipriano, D., Norris, L., & Olsen, S. (2010). Compassion fatigue and burnout: Prevalence among oncology nurses [Online exclusive]. *Clinical Journal of Oncology Nursing, 14*(5), E56–E62. doi:10.1188/10.CJON.E56-E62

Purnell, M.J., & Mead, L.J. (2007). When nurses mourn: Layered suffering. *International Journal for Human Caring, 11*(2), 47–52.

Qaseem, B., Shea, J., Connor, S.R., & Casarett, D. (2007). How well are we supporting hospice staff? Initial results of the Survey of Team Attitudes and Relationships (STAR) validation study. *Journal of Pain and Symptom Management, 34*, 350–358. doi:10.1016/j.jpainsymman.2007.06.003

Radziewicz, R.M. (2001). Self-care for the caregiver. *Nursing Clinics of North America, 36*, 855–869.

Raphael, B., & Wooding, S. (2004). De-briefing: Its evolution and current status. *Psychiatric Clinics of North America, 27*, 407–423. doi:10.1016/j.psc.2004.03.003

Saakvitne, K.W., & Pearlman, L.A. (1996). *Transforming the pain: A workbook on vicarious traumatization for helping professionals who work with traumatized clients.* New York, NY: W.W. Norton & Company.

Scholar, G. (2010). *Fit nurse: Your total plan for getting fit and living well.* Indianapolis, IN: Sigma Theta Tau International.

Sheets, V.R. (2001). Professional boundaries: Staying in the lines. *Dimensions of Critical Care Nursing, 20*(5), 36–40. doi:10.1097/00003465-200109000-00010

Sherman, D.W. (2004). Nurses' stress and burnout: How to care for yourself when caring for patients and their families experiencing life-threatening illness. *American Journal of Nursing, 104*(5), 48–56.

Skovholt, T.M., & Trotter-Mathison, M. (2011). *The resilient practitioner: Burnout prevention and self-care strategies for counselors, therapists, teachers, and health professionals* (2nd ed.). New York, NY: Routledge/Taylor & Francis Group.

Smith, P. (2009). *To weep for a stranger: Compassion fatigue in caregiving.* Mountain View, CA: Healthy Caregiving.

Notes

Stichler, J.F. (2009). Healthy, healthful, and healing environments: A nursing imperative. *Critical Care Nursing Quarterly, 32,* 176–188. doi:10.1097/CNQ.0b013e3181ab9149

Tariman, J.D. (2010). Where to draw the line? Professional boundaries in social networking. *ONS Connect, 25*(2), 10–13.

Tugade, M.M., & Fredrickson, B.L. (2004). Resilient individuals use positive emotions to bounce back from negative emotional experiences. *Journal of Personality and Social Psychology, 86,* 320–333. doi:10.1037/0022-3514.86.2.320

Wakefield, A. (2000). Nurses' responses to death and dying: A need for relentless self-care. *International Journal of Palliative Nursing, 6,* 245–251.

Walton, A.M.L., & Alvarez, M. (2010). Imagine: Compassion fatigue training for nurses. *Clinical Journal of Oncology Nursing, 14,* 399–400. doi:10.1188/10.CJON.399-400

Wenzel, J., Shaha, M., Klimmek, R., & Krumm, S. (2011). Working through grief and loss: Oncology nurses' perspectives on professional bereavement [Online exclusive]. *Oncology Nursing Forum, 38,* E272–E282. doi:10.1188/11.ONF.E272-E282

White, D. (2006). The hidden costs of caring: What managers need to know. *Health Care Manager, 25,* 341–347.

Zander, M., Hutton, A., & King, L. (2010). Coping and resilience factors in pediatric oncology nurses. *Journal of Pediatric Oncology Nursing, 27,* 94–108. doi:10.1177/1043454209350154

Recommended Reading

Adriaenssens, J., De Gucht, V., Van Der Doef, M., & Maes, S. (2011). Exploring the burden of emergency care: Predictors of stress-health outcomes in emergency nurses. *Journal of Advanced Nursing, 67,* 1317–1328. doi:10.1111/j.1365-2648.2010.05599.x

Cummings, G.G., Olson, K., Hayduk, L., Bakker, D., Fitch, M., Green, E., … Conlon, M. (2008). The relationship between nursing leadership and nurses' job satisfaction in Canadian oncology work environments. *Journal of Nursing Management, 16,* 508–518. doi:10.1111/j.1365-2834.2008.00897.x

Cuneo, C.L., Cooper, M.R.C., Drew, C.S., Naoum-Heffernan, C., Sherman, T., Walz, K., & Weinberg, J. (2011). The effect of Reiki on work-related stress of the RN. *Journal of Holistic Nursing, 29,* 33–43. doi:10.1177/0898010110377294

Hayes, C., Ponte, P.R., Coakley, A., Stanghellini, E., Gross, A., Perryman, S., … Somerville, J. (2005). Retaining oncology nurses: Strategies for today's nurse leaders. *Oncology Nursing Forum, 32,* 1087–1090. doi:10.1188/05.ONF.1087-1090

Latham, C.L., Hogan, M., & Ringl, K. (2008). Nurses supporting nurses: Creating a mentoring program for staff nurses to improve the work environment. *Nursing Administration Quarterly, 32,* 27–39. doi:10.1097/01.NAQ.0000305945.23569.2b

Notes

Rose, J., & Glass, N. (2008). Enhancing emotional well-being through self-care: The experience of community health nurses in Australia. *Holistic Nursing Practice, 22,* 336–347. doi:10.1097/01.HNP.0000339345.26500.62

Rushton, C.H., Reder, E., Hall, B., Comello, K., Sellers, D.E., & Hutton, N. (2006). Interdisciplinary interventions to improve pediatric palliative care and reduce health care professional suffering. *Journal of Palliative Medicine, 9,* 922–933. doi:10.1089/jpm.2006.9.922

Sabo, B.M. (2011). Compassionate presence: The meaning of hematopoietic stem cell transplant nursing. *European Journal of Oncology Nursing, 15,* 103–111. doi:10.1016/j.ejon.2010.06.006

Schluter, P.J., Turner, C., Huntington, A.D., Bain, C.J., & McClure, R.J. (2011). Work/life balance and health: The Nurses and Midwives e-cohort study. *International Nursing Review, 58,* 28–36. doi:10.1111/j.1466-7657.2010.00849.x

Internet Resources

American Holistic Nurses Association: www.ahna.org
Compassion Fatigue Awareness Project: www.compassionfatigue.org
Nurses Self Care: www.nursesselfcare.com
Schwartz Center for Compassionate Healthcare: www.theschwartzcenter.org

INDEX

ABOUT THE AUTHORS

Nancy Jo Bush, RN, MN, MA, AOCN®, received her master's in oncology nursing from the University of California, Los Angeles, and her master's in clinical psychology from Pepperdine University in Malibu, CA. She currently is an assistant clinical professor and lecturer in the graduate program in the School of Nursing at the University of California, Los Angeles. Bush received intern experience in the area of marriage, family, and child counseling while at the Wellness Community in Westlake, CA, and while in private practice at Counseling West in West Hills, CA. She is co-editor of the text *Psychosocial Nursing Care Along the Cancer Continuum* and the recipient of several honors from the Oncology Nursing Society, including being recognized as the Advanced Oncology Certified Nurse (AOCN®) of the Year in 2002 and delivering the Mara Mogensen Flaherty Memorial Lectureship in psychosocial oncology in 2010. Bush has published widely in the area of psychosocial nursing and is certified as a clinical nurse specialist and nurse practitioner in oncology.

Deborah A. Boyle, RN, MSN, AOCNS®, FAAN, received her master's degree with a focus in oncology nursing from Yale University. A long-tenured oncology nurse holding a variety of roles in both comprehensive cancer centers and community cancer programs, she is a frequent lecturer nationally and internationally and the author of more than 200 publications. Boyle was inducted into the American Academy of Nursing in recognition of her efforts in promoting increased awareness of advanced practice nursing and the psychosocial sequelae of cancer in patients and their families and for her advocacy on behalf of the special needs of cancer survivors and the elderly with cancer. She is the recipient of numerous honors from the Oncology Nursing Society, including delivering both the Schering Clinical Lectureship and Mara Mogensen Flaherty Memorial Lectureship and receiving awards for her contributions to the oncology nursing literature and the promotion of quality of life in patients and families facing cancer. She currently is the oncology clinical nurse specialist at the Chao Family Comprehensive Cancer Center at the University of California, Irvine.